I Sleep at Red Lights

I Sleep at Red Lights

a true story of life after triplets

Bruce Stockler

ST. MARTIN'S PRESS ✿ NEW YORK

www.stmartins.com

Library of Congress Cataloging-in-Publication Data

Stockler, Bruce.
    I sleep at red lights : a true story of life after triplets / Bruce Stockler.
        p.   cm.
    ISBN 0-312-31526-0
    1. Parenthood.   2. Triplets.   I. Title.

HQ755.8.S757   2003
649'.1—dc21

                                                    2003041413

First Edition: June 2003

10   9   8   7   6   5   4   3   2   1

For my mother, Carolyn Rosenblatt Stockler

CONTENTS

I Sleep at Red Lights

ONE

Seven Weeks

The ultrasound suite at New York Hospital is familiar, a bland and antiseptic box of a room with nothing special to steal our attention, no windows or magazines or glossy pharmaceutical company brochures to distract us from our anxiety.

Our son, Asher, was conceived here three years ago at the hospital's in-vitro-fertilization (IVF) clinic. We have undergone three failed IVF cycles since then, including two ectopic pregnancies, one of which went misdiagnosed in the emergency room and nearly killed my wife, Roni.

This is our last chance, I say to myself. I can't go through this anymore—the worrying, the waiting, the needles and injections and endless trips to obscure drugstores, the jumping when the phone rings, and, more than anything, the frantic 2:00 A.M. cab rides across Central Park to the ER. Not knowing what's wrong, if this is another bump in the road, the next agonizing end of a pregnancy, or a threat to Roni's life—the stress is too much.

We're lucky. We have a beautiful son. The boundaries of fertility, medical technology, probability, age, drug exposure, and our own fragile peace of mind cannot be pushed indefinitely.

Roni looks up from the examining table and smiles. I smile back.

Roni is panicking. She must be. She made the bed this morning, so I know she is upset. It has been at least a year since she made the bed. When she makes the bed, she is coming apart at the seams.

"Hi, honey," I say, stupidly. What do I say?

The ultrasound doctor enters the room. The blandly named Dr. Mills has generically handsome blond looks and a polite, regionally nonspecific speaking voice. He could be the product of the Greenwich WASP aristocracy, a preppy Jewish kid from Dallas or Tulsa, or an ambitious small-town Minnesota Lutheran.

"Good morning," Dr. Mills says without a smile. He fires up the aging computer workstation, types, then swivels in his chair, with a practiced minimum of effort and motion, to squirt conductive jelly onto the thin head of the ultrasound wand. This will be an internal ultrasound, not the tummy-top ultrasound so popular on TV shows.

We are at seven weeks. Roni and I have a chemical pregnancy, which is like a real pregnancy, with a dead bunny rabbit, but filtered through layers and layers of intrusive testing and probing, statistics and probabilities, maybes and wait-and-sees.

Seven weeks is a natural biological precipice, the period of greatest spontaneous abortion for all pregnant women. You may take a deep breath once you reach week number eight. We've been holding our breath for days now and we are dizzy from the exercise.

．　．　．

The ultrasound room is dark, lit only by the monochrome glow of the computer screen. Dr. Mills works the ultrasound wand slowly and wordlessly, with confident, fluid motions. There is the steady *beep, beep* of the imaging software and a *zoosh* as the backup drive fires and snaps a digital picture. But of what?

Roni is flat on her back. She can see the screen only by prying herself up off the examining table by the elbows and craning her neck to look through the valley of her splayed legs, planted wide apart in the stirrups. This must be the most difficult viewing position ever devised. Probably, I realize, this is by design—the clinic wants women supine, relaxed, and not thinking about it, which is preposterous.

The grainy black-and-white images are as cheesy as government hygiene films from the 1950s. I have watched dozens of ultrasounds, but still have no idea what I am seeing. The landscape of my wife's uterus remains an impenetrable mystery. I don't have the faintest idea what is going on in there.

Fifteen minutes pass by without a single word from Dr. Mills. He stops several times to replenish the conductive jelly. The machine beeps. The hard drive kicks in. The air is warm and stale with CPU exhaust.

I stare at the sonar readings of Roni's reproductive system. During Asher's pregnancy, I remember seeing the egg sac, a tiny white ring rising and falling on dark mountains of water. Now I see nothing but black, grainy emptiness, oceans of it.

We lost the pregnancy, I think. There's nothing there.

Beep. Zoosh. The computer is busy. Life is reduced to a palette of sound effects.

The doctor is recording the pathological evidence. What went wrong. Uterine this, morphology that. Chemicals. Hormone levels. Nature's cruel efficiency.

I stand in a corner behind Dr. Mills, a spiderweb tickling the back of my neck. My brain beams down thought waves into the doctor's cranium—*Say something, say anything, say some English words, you crazy silent medical bastard!*

Roni smiles at me, her eyes wet with fear.

I smile back, lying with every muscle in my face.

Time drags on mockingly. Without warning, Roni and I blurt out together:

"Okay!"

"What's happening?"

"Please say something!"

"Hello!?"

Our joint outburst does not affect Dr. Mills, who remains ignorant of the cosmological rarity of our convergent thinking.

Dr. Mills snaps more images, checks his files, then pushes his chair back. He diffidently removes his glasses and crosses his legs to reveal bare ankles and expensive tassel loafers.

"We are trained not to speak during the procedure, so we don't impart any false impressions," Dr. Mills says. This caution comes from isolated lawsuits across the country in which parents who assumed they were having a girl at fifteen weeks sued the hospital when the fetus sprouted a penis at twenty-six weeks, explains Dr. Mills, with a practiced monotone. This man is human tapioca pudding. My pulse aches in my throat.

Dr. Mills scrolls through the sequence of recorded images. "As you can see by this series, I detected three distinct embryonic structures. Each of them presents with an appropriate level of cardiovascular activity. A fourth site is also indicated, here, but is probably undergoing reabsorption into the uterine lining. . . ."

I stare at the computer screen. I do not understand.

"Could you say that again?" I hear a voice say. This is surprising, because I recognize the voice. It is my voice.

"Yes," Dr. Mills says. "I have outlined three egg sacs with excellent morphology. The first is here, along the top of the uterine wall. The second is here, just below it. The third is quite difficult to see, because it is actually implanted in tissue directly underneath the second, and the ultrasound cannot detect structures located . . ."

Roni looks over at me blankly.

"I still don't understand," I hear the voice say again.

Dr. Mills examines us with a slight tilt of his head. We are biological specimens, too, only larger and perhaps dangerous.

"I see . . . yes. Well. You are carrying triplets. They are in the seventh week of gestation. Seven weeks old."

Roni and I look at each other.

"Let me offer my official congratulations," Dr. Mills says, turning back to the computer. "Let's look at the egg sacs again. With triplets, the distribution of the embryos across the uterus is difficult . . ."

Roni and I stare at each other for a moment, then look around the room, lost and confused, like dogs dropped onto the surface of a strange and dogless planet.

The women in the IVF clinic waiting room stare at Roni. It is a customary ritual, a kind of uterus-to-uterus psychic friends network. Roni gazes over their heads, unblinking. She is pale and shivers from the arctic blasts of air conditioning.

We step onto the sidewalk outside New York Hospital. It is a Friday afternoon, a bright summer day, and we both squint horribly, blinded, after an hour in a dark room, by the harsh midday sun. The traffic on York Avenue and Sixty-eighth Street whizzes by carelessly.

"Are you going back to the office?" I say.

"Should we share a cab downtown?" Roni says.

"Maybe we should get something to eat," I say.

"Is it lunchtime?" she says.

We don't know what to do. We feel numb and soft, like frozen sticks of butter defrosting.

We share a cab downtown, holding hands across the backseat but looking out our own windows. Roni climbs out at Thirty-ninth and Third Avenue, waves good-bye, and wanders into Au Bon Pain. She looks back at me as the cab pulls away. In the crowded store she looks even tinier than her five-foot, 105-pound size. Why is she standing in Au Bon Pain? She doesn't drink coffee or eat pastries. Maybe they started selling soup for lunch, or Caesar salads with grilled chicken. Roni is a picky eater. She will eat the same lunch every day for a year.

The cab takes me across town but becomes gridlocked on Thirty-fourth Street, near Sixth Avenue, so I jump out and walk west to my office on Eighth Avenue. Midtown is crowded and noisy, like in those dystopian 1970s movies where Earth is overpopulated and the government has dissolved the Bill of Rights. My building is Five Penn Plaza, a tedious block-long building with a Blimpie's and a DMV office on the ground floor.

I am the editor-in-chief of a film magazine, a trade magazine read by directors, producers, animators, editors, and special-effects experts. I have been the chief editor for two years and was a senior editor the previous seven years. The job is enjoyable because I write about projects and artists I find the most interesting. I take a stack of VHS and ¾-inch cassettes into the conference room, where the tape decks are set up, and watch clips of TV commercials.

Dancing gasoline pumps, flying Listerine bottles, animated-clay celebrity boxing matches—I watch hundreds of tapes every week. Movies, TV shows, TV commercials: Everyone believes their creative project will transform the world. You can't put in the hours and not think it.

Harry, my technology writer, strolls in, eating a soggy vegetarian meatball sandwich, to remind me about our Monday meeting with Decker Computing to discuss their new rendering workstations. It will be a long meeting, full of flip charts, PowerPoint presentations, sales brochures, and white papers. They will discreetly inquire what kind of coverage they can expect. My job is to find a good reason to cover them while pretending we enjoy total editorial independence—which makes our coverage seem even more tantalizing. In the back of my mind, questions are starting to bubble up, but I have to call a man back about the latest developments in 3-D animated hair and fur.

Asher sleeps quietly in his Fisher Price car bed. It is 9:00 P.M. Friday night. After work I took Asher to Riverside Park and pushed him on the swings, then walked him through our regular play circuit—slide, play area, pigeon chasing.

We ate pizza and Italian ices. He rode around on my shoulders like the king of West 114th Street.

A stack of books—*Tom and Pippo*, *Oh My Oh My Oh Dinosaurs*, *Good Night Moon*—sits next to Asher's bed.

It has cooled outside, so I cover Asher with blankets from our bed, which he will invariably thrash to the floor. I don't know why I bother to cover him, but I always do, unless it is boiling hot in the apartment. Then I uncover him and throw open the windows. You are either boiling hot or freezing cold in New York. You can never be comfortable. You can never be just right.

Roni arrives home from work about 9:30 P.M. She is an attorney who works in corporate law, with a specialty in initial public offerings.

"Half day?" I say. This is an old joke. Her schedule is backbreaking—sixty, seventy, eighty hours a week, even more during a deal.

Roni throws her suit on the bed, changes into a big T-shirt, and goes to the bathroom. I remove the chicken, rice, and beans from the take-out bags. I pour seltzer and orange juice, fifty-fifty.

We eat dinner and watch TV in the den, taking turns with the remote control. We are each allowed one full cycle from Channel 2 through 99 before we switch. We both hate Friday nights because neither of us has a show on.

We eat quietly. Roni leafs through a magazine when it is my turn to flip.

"This is good chicken," I say.

"Yes. It is good chicken," Roni says.

We chew quietly for awhile. I pass the yellow rice and black beans.

"Is this the Brazilian chicken?" Roni asks.

"Yes," I say. "From Flor de Mayo." Flor de Mayo is one of our favorite take-out places, a Chino-Latino restaurant on 103rd Street and Broadway.

"We should save some for Asher," Roni says.

She's right. Asher loves the Brazilian chicken.

"Great idea," I say. "I'll save some chicken for Asher."

Roni finds a mystery show she recognizes on one of the public TV channels.

"Is that a good magazine?" I say.

"Yes," Roni says. "Antiques."

"Oh," I say. "I bet that's interesting."

The phone rings, but stops before the machine picks up.

"I wonder who that was," I say.

"They didn't leave a message," she says.

"It's spicy," I say. "The chicken."

"Right," she says.

"But not too spicy," I say.

"No, just spicy enough," Roni agrees.

"Sometimes I like it spicier, though," I say. "But sometimes I don't."

At 11:00 we watch a rerun of *Law and Order* on A&E, our favorite show, the cultural glue that binds us. We watch every new episode faithfully, at 10:00 P.M. Wednesday nights. We have seen every rerun many times and play a game when the rerun starts—Name the Perp.

"I miss Michael Moriarity," Roni says, during the commercial break.

"I know," I say. "Me too."

Roni puts her feet up on my lap and I squeeze her toes. We relax, comforted by the safe, familiar presence of our old friends in the Manhattan DA's office.

Later that night, I wake up to the sound of sawing. I look around, confused, then realize I have snored myself awake.

I check the clock. It is 2:19 A.M.

Now there is another noise, a clicking.

Click . . . click-click-click, goes the noise. It is creepy, this odd noise in the dead of night, and my adrenaline starts pumping.

Roni is not in the bed. She never leaves the bed, even to use the bathroom, unless she is sick. She must be chased out of bed in the morning with pointed sticks.

I find Roni in the kitchen, in the dark, sitting on the floor amid packing boxes, stacks of dishes splayed out around her, odds and ends dug up from the depths of storage. Drawers and cabinets lie open with junk overflowing everywhere, like entrails. Roni is typing on a labeling gun. Labels are everywhere and stuck to everything.

"Honey?" I say.

Roni does not acknowledge my presence. She squats on one knee, working furiously.

Click-click-click, goes the labeler.

"Honey?" I say.

". . . a full basement, because we can't keep living with boxes, like we're college students anymore—"

I sit down on the floor and try to catch Roni's eye. She stares down into her hands.

"Honey? Are you all right?" I say.

"I'll do a spreadsheet," she says. "Marla has a program that prints out color-coded labels. . . ."

The clicking continues. I see labels stuck to the floor: "kjJlillp" and "FFgnty."

I put my hand over hers to stop the labeler.

"Honey," I say. "Look at me."

Roni looks up at me, glassy eyed. She is traveling between distant galaxies, bouncing off dark matter, body surfing the invisible quantum force.

"You don't think God would play a joke on us, do you?" she says. "Give us three babies, then let something happen to them?" Her voice is quivering.

I hug her, but her body is stiff and unyielding.

"No," I say, with a conviction that surprises me. As soon as the words are out, I know this is true. This is not a religious belief, or faith, just an instinct.

"It's okay," I say. "It's almost eight weeks. We're going to be fine."

Something about my tone works. Roni puts down the labeler and closes the nearest box. We climb back into bed and spoon together, looking through the open French doors into the living room, where Asher is sleeping, his sweet face lit up by a mixture of moonlight and ambient city light.

"When I woke up, I thought maybe I had dreamed the whole day today, so I went to turn on the TV, to see what day it was," Roni says.

During our honeymoon in Italy, we saw a big Italian family at a restaurant in Florence, all the kids eating and talking and toasting each other. For a moment I imagined how much fun it would be to have a large family, but I never said anything to Roni. This was before we found out

Roni's fallopian tubes had been ruined, when babies were still just a matter of penciling in a time and place. I am drifting back to Tuscany, to bread soup and olive trees and red and orange leaves chasing our Fiat down empty country roads.

"Where are we going to live?" Roni says.

We are doubling, from three to six. I lift my head and look around the apartment.

With one bedroom and seven hundred square feet, that leaves about one hundred square feet per person, twice the size of an average prison cell. I think about our boxes, stacked everywhere and covered with dust, the closets jammed full of junk we have not seen in years, the bookshelves that boil over, and my stomach begins to turn with anxiety. I put my hand on Roni's stomach, spoon her closer to me, and try to fall asleep. As my eyes drift closed I see Asher turning in his sleep, his bedcovers thrashed to the floor.

TWO

The Big Family

Three. I run the idea over and over in my mind, but it hardly makes sense. Three new children sounds magical, biblical, Bladerunner-ish. One day soon I will wake up and discover three additional people living in my house. They will look like me, have my last name, and depend on me. It will be an invasion from a helpless and flatulent planet.

Twins are everywhere in New York City, thanks to the high-end fertility clinics that popped up like Korean nail salons. But triplets, quadruplets, and other megaplets are still a rare phenomenon, fodder for women's magazines and prime-time news shows.

Clearly, we have received a blessing of the highest order. I love my son deeply, more than my wife or even myself. More kids means more love. And more love is good.

After we learned that in-vitro fertilization and adoption were our only childbearing choices, we both secretly nurtured a wish for a big family. We never said a word about it, to avoid making the other feel guilty. Yet we both imagine a houseful of children, the roof bursting off in raucous cartoon puffs, Thanksgiving dinners blazing with revelry, a revolving front door of play dates and drop-ins and sleep-overs, snacks pouring out of kitchen cabinets like howitzer fire. Carolyn, my mom, has one younger sister, and Len, my dad, one younger sister. I have one younger brother, Roni one older sister. We come from a world of twos. To add three children will bump us up to four. We will double overnight.

Roni is watching the Prevue Channel, which I joke is her favorite show. I drag a laundry bag to the front door. It is 10:20 on Monday night, three days after the big news, which we have studiously ignored.

I talk to Roni from the hallway, which she hates. I am always talking and walking, she says, as if I'm trying to escape. In a thousand small ways husbands are always try-ing to escape.

Roni pops into the hallway and suddenly seems very small. She is petite and pale, with freckles and reddish blond hair, a Melanie Mayron type. Asher at birth was nine pounds and four ounces, a big old Caesarean like me. Big babies run on my side. The Stocklers and Rosenblatts (my mother's side of the family) don't grow tall but start out life with a bang.

I worry how Roni will carry three giant, barrel-chested, big-hipped babies to term. She gained twenty pounds with Asher. She can't gain sixty pounds with three babies or she might explode. I try hard not to think of all the horror and sci-fi movies littering my brain. What are the economies of scale in multiples gestation?

"Why are you looking at me like that?" Roni says.

I hold three fingers up. A flash of panic washes over her face and then she smiles.

"It's a miracle," I say.

"This is the part where the husband hugs the woman," Roni says. The fact that she says it causes me to hesitate. Even in moments of existential tenderness I manage to fail pathetically in my husbandly duties.

I spend Monday and Tuesday hiding in my office, hoping no one calls a staff meeting. My secret would cause flames of karmic anxiety to shoot out the back of my head, I worry, and set the Levelors on fire. How was I going to juggle the babies and Asher and six full-time editors and the art director and production manager and the freelancers and trips to New Orleans and L.A. and Silicon Valley and sneaking out for doctor's appointments and diaper shopping and taking over for the nanny when she calls in sick?

On Tuesday night I look around our unrenovated, ripped-up apartment, wondering how we can possibly live here. If we sublease the place and move out, we will have to fix it up. If we sell it, we will take a beating. But where will we go? How can we afford a bigger apartment when we are treading water with this albatross? Should we leave the city? I won't live in New Jersey and Roni won't live in Long Island or any of the other four boroughs. I've always wanted to live in the Arizona desert, or in northern California, or a dairy farm in Vermont, but I am a terrible creature of habit and I hate packing more than anything, except, possibly, unpacking.

"Let's not talk about it now," Roni says.

Denial is our executive strategy for the next two months. Friends and relatives are informed on a strict need-to-know basis, but otherwise we pretend nothing is different.

"Triplets?" my mom says. Her worry is as thick as electromagnetic interference.

"It's going to be just fine," I say.

"Triplets," my mom says.

I start laughing and she gets mad.

"Actually, we're having quads, but we decided to sell one to help amortize the cost," I say.

"You're terrible!" my mother says. She is laughing and crying. She is happy and sad, but mostly she is worried Asher and I will be swept away in the tidal wave of change. I reassure her and wonder if I am talking to myself.

Roni's mother takes the news more stoically.

"How are you going to pay for them?" Roni's mom says.

"One step at a time," Roni says.

At night, as Roni falls asleep, I keep an eye on her stomach, waiting for the sign that we can start planning for the lifestorm headed our way.

I am in Riverside Park at 112th Street, pushing Asher on the swings. He still enjoys the baby swings even though he graduated to the big-boy swings. It is the end of June and the park is full, with moms waiting patiently for spots.

"We have to let the other kids have a turn," I say, after five minutes.

"One more minute," Asher says.

As we leave I count three baby swings and four big-kid swings. Asher and I walk to the sandbox area as a gale of anxiety washes over me. How will I push Asher on the swing while managing three babies? How will I push four kids on four swings? How will I pay for four college educations? Will we need six cars when they are teenagers?

Asher plays contentedly in the sandbox. He holds up a shovel of sand and pretends to eat it.

"No eating sand!" I say, pretending to be angry. When Asher was ten or eleven months old he sometimes ate sandbox sand. Now we share a joke about it. He's not even three yet but comments ironically on his infancy.

I enjoy documenting every twist and turn in Asher's development. I remember with photographic clarity the first time he said "Daddy," the first time he slid down the big-kid slide alone, his first taste of falafel.

How will I provide this level of attention to four kids? Fatherhood is a service industry and I am growing from one to four clients without any additional resources.

I study Asher's sweet little face. I know what he is thinking or feeling or even which way he is going to run just by reading his face. How will I meet his needs? How will he get our attention over three screaming babies?

"He's going to have three best friends for the rest of his life," Roni says, when I confess my anxiety that night. Like a sudden change in the wind, Roni is the positive one and I the negative.

I lie down on the floor and watch Roni clip Asher's toenails, which are so thin they look like cellophane. This genetic nod to Roni's side of the family gives her great relief when she grimaces at my thick, yellowing werewolf toenails.

Roni works carefully and with great tenderness. She clips Asher's toenails when he is sleeping because he cries when he is awake, not out of pain but fear. Roni prides herself on keeping Asher's nails trimmed and his clothes as unwrinkled as possible, given that neither of us know how to operate an iron. She spends a lot of time buying him nice shirts on sale, taking him for noninvasive haircuts, buying him toys that stimulate and challenge him. When he was a baby, she spent hours reading the nutrition labels on traditional baby food, and then organic baby food, and she became so discouraged by the mediocrity of the ingredients that she began making her own baby food for him.

"How are we going to spend time with Asher when we're changing three diapers, running to the store for formula, doing eight million loads of laundry?" I say.

"We'll do things together," Roni says. "You'll read a book to Asher and all the kids will listen." She is very calm and confident about this, which makes me wonder if she is cruising on a higher spiritual plane or riding a dangerously unbalanced hormonal riptide.

I can't imagine how this Musketeerish, all-for-one scenario will fall together. Then I feel guilty because across the crystal-blue seas of our awesome blessing spreads the oil slick of my anxiety.

Later that night I sit with Asher as he settles into bed. I relish the quiet time sitting and talking about his day, singing stupid made-up songs, answering his volleys of questions, and watching him fall asleep with his little hands entwined with mine. Sometimes I feel in danger of becoming a male version of those hypervigilant, affection-starved moms in Riverside Park who smother their kids with baby talk and too many sweaters and frantic yelps over every cough and playground tussle and skinned knee. They are everywhere in the city with their bug-eyed woogly-woos and who's-the-bests and you're-so-specials, lost inside the existential wonder of their child.

How will Asher react to having three little brothers and/or sisters? How will he adapt to losing his status, his space, his time with me and Roni, his sense of being that special little man in our lives? What will it be like for a three-year-old to have the rug yanked out from under him and his dizziness explained away as good fortune?

I consider myself mature and cultured, but in fact am highly inflexible and cling to the comfortable and the familiar. If Roni and I plan on dinner and a movie, and in the elevator she announces her intention to go dancing instead, I tilt like an old pinball machine at this berserk shift in the universe. "That's not the plan!" I say, as if dancing instead of dinner represents a logistical nightmare on the order of moving D-day.

Will Asher be flexible as we shake his world upside down? Or will he be like me, freak out, and develop nervous tics? I have been rubbing my forehead with my fingertips since I was a kid, and have a slight discoloration on one side of my head, which, when I am really anxious, worry has turned into a melanoma.

From the day he was born, I wanted Asher to have a peaceful inner life. With triplets running in screaming circles in his outer life, I wonder how this goal is even possible now.

"We have enough love to go around," Roni says. "Love is like water. It expands to fill whatever space needs to be filled."

But water is inelastic, I say. It doesn't expand or contract unless it turns to gas or ice. What if our love turns into gas and floats away into the atmosphere? Our water supply will be divided by a factor of four, leaving us a dire water shortage . . .

Roni is irritated by my theatrical analogies and metaphors. "You need to worry about *your wife*," Roni says. "You need to worry about how you're going to pay attention to me. Come here and rub my feet."

"There's going to be a seventy-five percent reduction in foot rubbing," I say.

"You used to rub my feet all the time," she says, moaning softly.

I think about making a joke, and then think better of it. I take tiny steps forward in the husband-improvement department, only to make sudden, Olympic, backward leaps.

At work on Monday I fax Roni a muddy photocopy of my hand with three fingers held up. I hide three cookies in her briefcase. I put three flowers in a vase. Teasing her is a childish but effective way to release my own anxiety.

Roni begins to show in early July. This prompts stage two in the disinformation campaign—close friends learn the truth, while casual friends, co-workers, and acquaintances are told only that Roni is pregnant, which I rationalize as a technical truth. We feel compelled to cover up our situation because excess scrutiny will raise our stress levels and turn us into objects of needless office speculation.

Roni's ob-gyn, Dr. Rivera, calmly debriefs us on the perils of carrying triplets. "Have you considered selective reduction?" Dr. Rivera asks, point-blank, after pronouncing Roni healthy at her twelve-week exam.

We are stunned. Dr. Rivera is the warmest, smartest, most accomplished doctor we have ever met. She is in her early thirties, short and thin, attractive, and radiates a warm, omnipotent glow. With all the worries and minor complications of Asher's C-section, Dr. Rivera stood steadfast and strong and guided us to a safe landing. I trust Roni's life and the lives of the three babies to her completely. Dr. Rivera is like a god to me.

Dr. Rivera sees the shocked look on our faces and apologizes. She is ethically and legally bound to inform us of the risks of a multiple pregnancy. With Roni's age, forty-one, her small physical size and general condition (very little exercise, great mental stress), plus the inherent risk factors for triplets, our chance of facing complications is very high compared to a singleton birth. Even reducing from triplets down to twins shaves 40 or 50 percent off our risk factor for losing all three babies.

"We're not killing any of the babies," Roni says.

"Not a chance," I say.

"Now we have to talk about amniocentesis," Dr. Rivera says.

Without looking at Roni I signal our negative vote. Amnio poses anywhere from a .5 percent to 2 percent risk per baby of causing spontaneous abortion. We have to multiply that number by three, since Roni will face three separate needles. That means up to a 6 percent risk of killing our babies just to check for genetic problems. This is the first step down the long road to discretionary, à la carte genetic selection.

"We're just going forward, doing whatever we can to stay safe," Roni says.

"That brings up points three and four," says Dr. Rivera.

I hold my breath as Dr. Rivera explains that Roni must go into enforced bed rest. Depending on a variety of factors, she will need anywhere from ten to twenty weeks of bed rest.

"What do you mean by bed rest, *exactly?*" says Roni.

"We'll discuss that when the time is right," says Dr. Rivera.

"But I'll be able to work on the computer—" Roni says.

Dr. Rivera looks at me. Women are always looking at me in this way—What are you going to do about this? Do you see what is going on here?

How did I get appointed to this intergender ambassadorship? When Asher was born, Roni fought with a dozen hospital people, all the way up to the hospital administrator, to stay off the bedpan, even after the epidural. All the hospital brass looked at me for help. Roni is a lawyer who hates to follow the rules.

"I'm not getting involved with the master negotiator," Dr. Rivera says to me. "You're going to be in charge of her bed rest."

"He's not in charge of anything," Roni says.

"Last item," Dr. Rivera says: "the cerclage."

I look at Roni. She didn't mention this.

"Which is French for . . ." I say.

"We sew the cervix shut with surgical sutures," Dr. Rivera says. "It prevents the cervix from dilating prematurely."

My testicles retreat up into the safety of my abdomen and close the door behind them. This procedure sounds like Roni will be sewn shut like a Thanksgiving turkey, an image I vow never to share.

"When?" I say.

"Before bed rest begins," Dr. Rivera says.

"I just want the babies to be healthy," Roni says.

"Then we'll take this one step at a time," Dr. Rivera says. Dr. Rivera smiles at me. After several years it finally strikes me that Dr. Rivera is one smoking-hot woman, as much for her capabilities and intelligence as her slim, dark good looks. I don't share this information, either.

We rent a small house for the summer in Westport, Connecticut, a picture-perfect town on the Long Island Sound. The plan is to escape out there on weekends and ignore the arrival of the triplets in a more luxurious setting.

Roni is so exhausted that she hardly notices we are on a weekend getaway. We drive up to Connecticut late Friday night and Roni sleeps and watches TV almost the entire weekend. I don't even think she knows which direction the beach is. She's not a sun person, anyway, but I push her to read or cook or garden before she loses any more of her orbital path.

I take Asher to the town beach every day. We splash in the still waters of the Sound and study the beach houses and the sailboats and the far-off spine of Long Island. We build wobbly sand castles and bury our feet in the dark, wet sand. The public beach has a large open playground, which I chase Asher across and up and down for hours. We take refuge in the snack shack, where Asher orders french fries and easily manipulates me into buying him cherry ices.

In the late afternoon we pick up Roni and cruise around Westport. Roni antiques a bit, wanders around the organic supermarket and shows Asher all kinds of exotic and overpriced items. We eat brick-oven pizza.

One day I sit on the sand and watch Asher dig. My face is glowing. Peals of Asher's laughter and the calls of the gulls ring around me. The hot sun bakes me into a buttery trance, and the blue sky, the warmth of Asher's hand as he pulls me across the wooden gangplank of the play area, the sudden sweet smell of salt—for a few moments I feel as if we have stepped through a doorway into another place. I try to lock this moment into my mind so I can recall it in times of stress.

One afternoon, as we play croquet with plastic mallets and balls, we tell Asher that Mommy is going to have three babies. Asher whacks a few balls around and thinks about this.

"My babies," he says.

We will take care of the babies together, we say. He will be our helper and the three of us will have these three babies as our group project.

"But Daddy changes the diapers," Asher says. I tell Asher he can help me change the diapers and he looks at me like I am a lunatic. It's the same look Roni gives me.

That night I wake up in a clammy sweat and walk outside to cool off. I listen to the waves and let pictures from my childhood in the rough smoky waves of Atlantic City jumble around in my head. I crash toward the beach in my red raft; my brother Paul shivers in the cold tangy water; I huff for air as I climb through the storm front of foam and water for the surface; my mom sits on a beach chair squinting possessively after us. The ocean has always been an embracing place, and I float along on these memories until I realize we are on Long Island Sound. There is no great ocean shimmering out beyond the darkness, just a flat, up-scale pond. A metal tang of disappointment fills my mouth. The sound of the waves is only the wind in the trees.

It is not just rearranging our life that worries me. We have not discussed the deal in months now, and it hangs out there in the air between us. Roni has refrained from saying anything, but she is thinking about it, and her silence unnerves me.

Our deal is that Roni earns two-thirds of the household income and I am the caregiver. I change Asher's diapers and catch his vomit in my hands and wake up early in the morning with him and jump up in the middle of the night when he cries out. When Rosetta, the baby-sitter, is sick or takes her daughter to school or the doctor, I use up a vacation day. When Asher lost the little plastic cup he carried everywhere as his magical comfort object, I turned the apartment upside down until it was discovered.

Asher and I are so close that we are like our own little country. This is good for us but leaves Roni out in the cold, stuck on a guest visa. When Asher falls on the playground or wakes at night he cries out for Daddy. When Roni scoops him up, he struggles away to reach for me. I make a face at Roni as if to say, Isn't it funny how he is such a daddy's boy, and Roni makes a face back, as if to say, Oh, that son of yours, but I know how deeply this betrayal hurts.

Roni wants more time at home with Asher. She has been working like a dog for ten years and deserves a break. But she is also pushing to make partner at her law firm because she is a tough, thorough, reliable bulldog of a lawyer and demands the recognition and reward she deserves.

My journalism career will never approach Roni's salary yield as a lawyer. I would need to make a leap to another field—public relations or marketing—and as a senior person to boot, where I will compete with people who have ten to fifteen years more experience. Most headhunters won't even handle magazine editors—it's a nepotistic business, so why bother—and the one headhunter who takes me on sends me for a job interview at *Black Enterprise*, a magazine for black professionals. Not good. We have gone deeply into debt to pay for the in-vitro cycles and cannot afford to lose Roni's income now. Meanwhile, I am under pressure to travel with the sales guys in northern California, to hit up the new software and hardware clients. But when I leave town and Roni works till 1:00 in the morning, who will take care of Asher and three babies? Rosetta has her own daughter. Roni's mother can manage Asher, but not four kids. Our future is wide open and uncertain. The chicken-and-egg question of whether our marital role reversal is an accident of economics or a natural outgrowth of our basic natures will wait for a quieter time.

I am editing copy in my office, the phone ringing constantly. Finally, the receptionist buzzes and says Roni has been trying to reach me.

"My side hurts," she says.

"Which side?" I say. It's a stupid question, really, unless she's having appendicitis. It is late July now and Roni is about fourteen weeks pregnant.

"Does it hurt like you have gas or hurt like you have to go to the emergency room?" I say.

"It hurts," Roni says.

Roni is physically tough, tougher than most men, and never complains about pain. She has dental work done, drilling and root canal, without anesthetics. We have a problem. I tell Roni to head straight to the New York Hospital/Cornell emergency room on York Avenue and Seventy-first Street. I call Rosetta and warn her we might be late. I tell the people in my office that Roni got sick at work. The way I haul ass out of there is guaranteed to raise suspicion.

I find Roni in triage. Because she is pregnant, her wait in the emergency room was only a few minutes. Soon we are up on the eighth floor maternity ward. Roni's pain level is increasing dramatically—she is crushing my fingers and is moaning out loud.

"Get Dr. Rivera!" Roni says.

Dr. Rivera is somewhere between home and hospital, unreachable. Despite the attention around us, very little is done to actually diagnose Roni. It dawns on me that no one wants to touch a woman pregnant with triplets.

I demand to talk to the chief resident.

"I need something for the pain!" Roni says.

I don't know what to think. An ectopic pregnancy? She had both fallopian tubes removed after the last ectopic, so I don't think this can be another ectopic. But I don't know. I argue that we need the chief resident immediately, but this is not happening. I am stuck in a hard place between Roni's bossy panic and the hospital's bovine intransigence.

A fetal heartbeat monitor is attached and the fetal heart-beats appear normal. But Roni's blood pressure and pulse are soaring from the pain.

Another forty-five minutes goes by and nothing changes. "Goddamn it! Something is wrong!" Roni yells. One of the nurses tells Roni to keep her voice down.

"You can leave now," I tell the nurse. "No one tells my wife to quiet down when she's in pain and pregnant and no one is helping us!"

"I'm not going anywhere," the nurse says.

"Go read the patient's bill of rights!" I say.

I argue with the chief nurse. "You need to do something," I say. "My wife cut the tip of her finger off with a knife and didn't complain. She's not a whiner. *There's something wrong here and you people aren't doing anything.*"

They are monitoring Roni and the babies and will not do anything invasive until Dr. Rivera can be reached. They won't give pain medication because it will cross the uterine wall. She would need general anesthesia.

Another hour goes by. Roni screams at me to do something. The chief resident is monitoring the situation, I am told.

"From where—his summer home in Provence!" I say.

"Sarcasm isn't going to help," the chief nurse says.

"Doing nothing isn't helping!" I say.

Finally Dr. Rivera is reached on her cell phone. She instructs the staff to give Roni a small dose of Valium, which should be safe for the babies. From Roni's symptoms, Dr. Rivera thinks she has a kidney stone.

"Gee, that Valium—is that an experimental drug?" I say to the chief nurse.

Roni is given an ultrasound by one of the doctors from the in-vitro clinic who was reached by page. "We think she has a small kidney stone in her right kidney," the IVF doctor tells us. We have been in the hospital almost four hours now.

"And?" I say.

"It's very small, but it looks like it's getting ready to pass into the ureter, so it's pressing against the end of the kidney, which is why it's so painful," the IVF doctor says.

"So what are you going to do?" Roni says.

"We'll have to wait until it passes," the IVF doctor says.

Roni looks at me. I have no idea what to do or say,

except quietly pray for invisibility. I tell them we expect to see Dr. Rivera the second she hits the hospital.

Roni is given a low-dose Valium drip and her pain mercifully recedes. Roni pees into a cup with a filter, although the stone is probably too small to catch.

When Dr. Rivera makes her appearance we unload—the waiting, the hands-off approach, the rude nurses. Dr. Rivera has heard it all before, and probably worse, but expresses the right amount of sympathy to calm Roni down. The bad news is that Roni is now more likely to develop future kidney stones.

Some people take their kidney stones home in a specimen jar filled with alcohol. We take home a bill for $1,800. I stare at the bill in shock. The only way I could make $1,800 in a day would be to fake my own death and collect the insurance.

Roni was forbidden to eat in case she required surgery, so we stop for chicken kebabs and mujadara at the Lebanese restaurant near our apartment. By the time we walk in the door and hug Asher it feels as if we have been gone for a week. As we go to sleep that night, I feel we have dodged another bullet.

THREE

Bribing the Gynecologist

Ilsa, our tiny, ninety-something next-door neighbor, who blasts polka music through our adjoining living room wall at the oddest hours of the day and night, stares at Roni's stomach with utter confusion. We just told Ilsa that Roni is four months pregnant. Ilsa is examining Roni and doing the math.

Ilsa has memory problems, is on the paranoid side, has lost most of her hearing and eyesight, but has lived a full life, and the stomach she sees in front of her does not look like the stomach of a woman who is four months pregnant.

"Are you sure it's four months?" Ilsa says in her hard German accent. "These doctors sometimes make terrible mistakes!" Ilsa looks up anxiously at me.

It is the end of August. Roni is exhausted and looks due any day now. Her breasts are swollen tremendously. She is starting to look like a Macy's balloon that is having trouble staying afloat. When I look at Roni, I try to erase the anxiety from my mind, and visualize the Bonneville Salt

Flats and sheets of antarctic ice. I don't want to give her any reason to worry. It's all smooth, it's all good and solid and harmonious.

"What are you thinking?" Roni says.

"Oh, nothing," I say.

The end of the summer makes me melancholy. My days and nights with Asher were idyllic, filled with adventures like agitating the sandwich-stealing seagulls, insulting the groceries in the organic superstore, hunting for crabs in the rocks, digging in the wet sand with coffee cups. Asher's old routine of tumbling classes, music classes, and play dates feels anticlimactic.

In mid-September Roni is admitted for her cerclage on a Friday afternoon. I can't even think about this procedure without feeling dizzy. We are back home within hours. I wait on Roni hand and foot as she naps and moans all weekend, thankful I am a man.

Roni is bored with her condition and one night I find her brandishing the Mikita router—an old birthday present from me—to work on a new built-in shelf for the den.

"Maybe we should just watch TV," I say.

"Are you saying I'm incapacitated?" Roni says.

The problem with being a husband is that any question, no matter how innocent, can be a trick question.

"Uh, no, you looked a little tired?" I say.

"Oh, I look a little tired *today*, when I worked ten hours, but not yesterday, or the day before—you weren't worried about me *then*," Roni says.

This is the hormones talking. God only knows what is going on in her bloodstream hour to hour. But just because they are hormones doesn't mean they don't feel morally justified.

"I was worried about you then but I'm a little more worried now so I decided to say something, in terms of the being tired, and maybe taking a break, to help stave off more tiredness, and preserving, uh . . ." I say. "Uh, your energy?"

"Maybe you don't *like* the other bookshelf," she says.

"I love my bookshelf!" I say.

"Then why is all this crap stuffed in here?" she says, pointing to the books and papers and videotapes and odds and ends.

Now is not the time to remind her that the crap in evidence is miscellaneous junk I have been trying to toss out for years, a process she has filibustered with a final-review-of-junk power she refuses to exercise.

"Maybe we can clean it up a little bit," I say. I am ready to run out of the room with my head in a bag.

"No, I'm tired," Roni says, sitting down and putting her hands on her belly. Her eyes are droopy. She asks about Asher's day. I put her feet up and rub them and she falls asleep with a smile on her face. She breathes heavily now, with a slight wheeze. The babies are beginning to push on her diaphragm.

Nicky, my boss, finishes an extremely loud phone call with an advertiser as I wait in his blond-wood office. Nicky loves the film industry. He loves talking to the old videotape guys and selling ad space, and considers the magazine his family. He is a natural publisher, except for his sometimes Hunnish people skills. I lost my two best writers in the last two years, each one over a requested pay raise of $10,000 a year. Each writer cost us $20,000 or $25,000 more to replace. But that is how it works in business. The sanctity of the chain of command is more important than the battle logic on the ground.

I have withheld our news to the people in my office for months. Everyone else in our lives knows, but my office is small and clannish and I am the only one with young children. The gossip will be intense and I will be pinned down under a microscope.

Nicky gets off the phone and smiles at me. "Bosco!" he booms. Nicky maintains pet names for people. We chitchat for a few minutes and then I tell him Roni and I are having triplets.

Nicky's face hardens. His wide Yosemite Sam mustache flops down as if he has been shot in the foot.

"Really," Nicky says.

My face and ears burn as if someone rubbed habañero peppers on them. I don't know what to say. "We're very lucky," I blurt out, to fill the awkward silence.

"Huh," Nicky says.

Nicky's phone rings and he looks over at it with relief. "I have to grab this. Let's talk later," Nicky says.

I stomp back to my office with Nicky's voice booming behind me. I do not tell Roni or anyone else about this conversation because I worry I will pick up a phone or a snow globe and heave it at Nicky's head if he says anything sarcastic. A few days later we are discussing new business and Nicky says I should work half days to stretch out my transition back to a normal work schedule. Several times over the next few weeks I walk into Nicky's office when he is with the East Coast sales guy, Walter, and their conversation snaps shut.

.   .   .

We are in Dr. Rivera's office again. It is early October. I am continually fighting off the fear of an emergency, so Dr. Rivera's office has become a sanctuary.

"Hi, honey!" I say, waving at Roni, slumped on the examining table. She refuses to put on the dressing gown. She hides under her long, baggy T-shirt.

Roni stares at me. My idiotic cheerfulness is grating on her nerves. She likes Dr. Rivera but is anxious about further restrictions. I don't want her to resent her pregnancy, because it is the calm before the storm, and she needs to enjoy it.

Roni is six months pregnant and looks twelve. She is starting to have trouble walking because her swollen stomach and breasts caravan out far in front of her.

Dr. Rivera gives Roni a sonogram and a short internal exam to check on the cerclage. I hide in the back of the room, proofreading medical supply boxes.

"Everything looks good. I'll give you one week, and then you're on bed rest until you deliver," Dr. Rivera says, staring at me.

"What I was thinking—" Roni begins.

"Tell her to save the negotiating for the clients," Dr. Rivera tells me. "You're going to rent a fetal heartbeat monitor and get this prescription filled."

"I think I can decide what's best," Roni says.

"Yes, you can," Dr. Rivera says. "That's why you chose me." Dr. Rivera has delivered three or four sets of triplets, she is conservative, and she does not fool around.

Dr. Rivera wants Roni on fifteen weeks of bed rest, from week twenty or twenty-one until the scheduled C-section date of thirty-six weeks. Old-fashioned, regular babies are born at forty weeks. Twins are delivered at thirty-eight weeks. Triplets are delivered at thirty-six weeks because the placenta deteriorates so much faster and can't support the babies.

"Let's discuss what you mean by 'bed rest,' " Roni says. "Exactly."

Dr. Rivera fixes me with that steady gaze. "You will stay in bed or on a couch with your legs and feet up," Dr. Rivera says. "You will get up to go to the bathroom. You can walk for a few minutes a day to prevent your muscles from getting too weak."

Dr. Rivera patiently reviews the dangers of bringing triplets to term at the age of forty-one. Roni risks premature contractions, preterm labor, rupturing her cerclage, preeclampsia, and a host of other complications, including serious threats to her own life.

But it is difficult to accept fifteen weeks of sitting in bed, especially when you can't find a comfortable position. Roni is already having trouble sleeping. She suffers from heartburn and acid reflux, she can't sleep on her sides, and eats only a few bites of food at a time. She is on track to gain 50 pounds on her 110-pound frame, all in her stomach.

Dr. Rivera offers some strategies for sleeping and fighting heartburn and keeping her stomach from feeling full.

"But what am I going to do?" Roni says. "In bed?"

Dr. Rivera looks at me.

"We should look at this like a kind of special vacation," I say. "You can read books, work on your invention ideas, make things for Asher—"

"A vacation is Italy and bread soup and leaves falling," Roni says. "Not fifteen weeks of watching you asking me if I'm okay every ten seconds."

"You've always wanted time off from work," I say.

"They could fire me," Roni says.

"You two discuss this," Dr. Rivera says. "But I mean what I said. I want you to rest. No work, no phones, no faxes or email. The worst thing for you right now is mental stress. Stress is one of the primary factors for premature labor."

"I'm stressed out thinking about sitting in bed for fifteen weeks," Roni says.

Dr. Rivera gives me a look and leaves.

"Listen," I say. "Dr. Rivera says—"

Roni tells me to consider her day. I will leave the apartment at 9:00 A.M. for work. Asher leaves at 9:30 with Rosetta. Who will take care of Roni for the eight or nine hours until I get home? How is she going to secure her lunch? Her questions stop here, but mine continue: What happens if someone knocks on the door? What if she can't find the phone? We haven't planned for her to be abandoned all day.

"Don't worry," I lie. "I'll figure it out." Meanwhile I worry about the phone or the electricity or the pilot light going out. What if she has bleeding? The panic rises up in my stomach like a hot ulcer, so I change the subject to dinner. Roni says her heartburn is killing her. Dinner can wait until I find her a jumbo bottle of chewable antacid.

We convert the small den into a second bedroom, because the homemade bed in the master bedroom is too high. Roni built our bed based on a design from an antique Italian postcard. The bed has two-by-fours for legs with finials on top and a simple headboard and footboard. She cut the wood, drilled the holes, sawed the slats. But she never trimmed down the two-by-fours, so the bed stands waist height—for me—way too high for Roni. When Asher was a baby and came into bed with us, I had nightmares about him rolling off the edge of the bed and disappearing. Roni would need a freight elevator to get in and out of her bed now.

So we sleep in the TV room/home office/den/pregnancy room on the old futon couch, where she spends the rest of the day, imprisoned. She can't sleep because the babies press against her organs. She is short of breath. Her favorite foods cause terrible indigestion, reducing her diet to crackers, chicken soup, bits of boiled chicken, soft rolls. She drinks water, apple juice and flat ginger ale. Sometimes I walk into the den and see Roni slouching miserably, trapped in the dual prison of her body and our crumbly apartment, and the sight is so sad that I burst out in nervous, honking funeral laughs.

"It's not funny!" Roni says.

I curl up next to her and hug her, and tell her how sorry I am, how proud I am, how happy and excited I am. We will have a whole rock band, nearly half a softball team, two sides of a volleyball team, right in our own house.

"This is all your fault," she says.

"I know," I say. "Everything is my fault."

Roni is beyond huge and into the archaic and obscure Scrabble-level adjectives. By mid-October only the slightest hint of her belly button remains. It looks like a melted circle of plastic glued onto a balloon. Veins spider out across the moonscape of her stomach.

Roni taps me on the shoulder.

"I can't sleep," she says.

Leaning back on a mound of five pillows to keep her propped up and deter acid reflux, she towers over me. It is 4:30 in the morning.

"There's nothing on TV," Roni says.

"Read your book," I say.

"It's stupid," she says. "Do you want to play cards?"

Asher will be up in two to three hours. I feel badly for her, but I have not been sleeping well under this new routine, either—the lights on, the TV on, Roni readjusting her pillows every two minutes and moaning constantly, the sound of crackers being crunched with agonizing slowness, bits of cheese sliding down the pillow and into the crack of my neck, and Roni, always awake and hovering, like a grouchy and castle-bound vampire.

"Okay, let's play cards," I say. I can fall asleep playing cards. Maybe she won't notice.

"Do we have cards?" Roni says. In this room alone the cards could be in any one of three hundred hiding places. I get out of bed and poke around.

"As long as you're up, can I have a piece of cheese?" Roni says.

She nibbles on her cheese and says she intends to work at home, in direct violation of Dr. Rivera's orders. I object, but she cuts me off. "Do you know how stressed out I will be having nothing to do, and worrying if I will still have a job?" Roni says.

I give up. Roni may be obstinate and strong-willed, but she knows what makes her stressed out more than anyone else. And she earns two-thirds of our income, so she will have to skate us, big belly and all, across the thin ice of our financial stability.

. . .

In a few more weeks, Roni's feet and ankles start to swell up. She is in constant discomfort, exhausted and bored out of her mind.

Roni misses the old office gossip, even though she has become the subject, as rumors circulate about her size and possible complications. Some of the lawyers resent her taking a long leave of absence. Like any business that prides itself on its family values, her firm is full of intrigue.

Asher loves to pull up Roni's shirt and examine her belly. Roni's midsection is more exciting than a ride at an amusement park. The babies are especially active at night, and after 9:00 P.M. her stomach comes alive, the skin flexing this way and that, like a rubber bag full of angry cats.

Asher has many questions: Where will the babies sleep? What games can they play? What is their favorite TV show? But his attention is short-lived and he moves on to more pressing two-year-old concerns, such as why we can't call Christopher Robin on the phone. He is not worried about the arrival of the babies.

Roni looks forward to the twenty-six-week ultrasound, her first venture outside in four weeks. She leans on me in the hallway, keeping one hand under her belly, surprised by the gravitational pull. One of the neighbors waits for the elevator with us, her eyes nervously glued to Roni's stomach.

Outside in the shivering cold Roni feels energized. Normally she is always cold and I am always hot, but now, her body overheated by four metabolisms, she is running hot and feels great.

Roni is frighteningly skinny. She is losing weight in her legs, rear end, arms and face. Every calorie is funneled directly to the babies. Her stretch pants hang loosely around her and her swollen ankles stand out against her pale, dry, skinny legs. From certain angles she looks anorexic.

Roni wants to walk but is too tired. I lean her against the railing outside our building and run up to Broadway to catch a yellow cab. The cab circles down 113th Street and back up our block and pulls up to the building, but Roni is gone. I jump out, worried she has fallen down and rolled to the curb like a beer keg, but I find her inside the building, inspecting a marble-refinishing job in the lobby.

"Let's go, little doggy," I say. Roni is easily distracted, like a puppy dog. In the cab I tell the driver to go slowly—very, very slowly.

"Okay, boss," the driver says, sarcastically, until he throws a glance at Roni in the rearview mirror and his eyeballs shoot out of his head.

Sensory deprived for weeks, Roni bursts with information overload. She points out new stores and awnings and architectural details about buildings we have previously failed to notice. Winter-scarred Central Park seems like the gardens of Paris.

At New York Hospital's in-vitro clinic, the women in the waiting room regard Roni with reactions ranging from desperate baby lust to panic. Thought bubbles literally burst in the air around her. We check in here and then go down the first floor to see Dr. Rivera.

"Looking good," Dr. Rivera says. Roni might be getting a little anemic, so Dr. Rivera orders a blood work-up.

"I'm dying of boredom," Roni says. "I can't sleep. I'm eating one of those jumbo bottles of Tums every week."

Dr. Rivera tells Roni to sleep on her right side, a pillow between her legs, and pillows under her stomach to support the babies. But there is not much else to do. The babies are growing and her internal organs have nowhere to go.

"Watch the travel channel and pick out a vacation," Dr. Rivera says.

I look at Dr. Rivera with a sense of panic. Vacation?

That night Roni makes me promise two weeks in Tuscany if she makes it to thirty-six weeks. I can't comprehend who will watch three squalling infants while we tromp through olive groves, but that is a stomachache for the future.

A week later we are back at the IVF clinic to discuss the ultrasounds, which we assume are normal.

"We found some areas of concern," says the IVF doctor. He introduces the staff geneticist. We are seized with surprise. The geneticist explains that two of the babies exhibit markers for genetic defects. The second baby also has an enlarged right kidney.

These markers do not translate directly into possible birth defects. The cyst on Baby B's neck is something that usually resolves itself before birth, but the fact of its detection signifies an increased risk of birth defects, especially Down's syndrome. So two of the babies have increased risks for birth defects. The staff wants to do more invasive testing, including amnio. My head is spinning with surprise, anxiety—with anger. Enough is enough.

"No amnio," Roni says.

"No amnio," I say.

I press the doctors to explain "increased risk" but the answers are not definite. We might have a 20 or 30 percent higher risk than average for Roni's age group. It could even be higher. Or lower. Prenatal genetic testing is still inexact.

Roni and I are in shock, but we know one thing—we will not take any steps that jeopardize the babies' health, even with the risk of Down's syndrome. The staff leaves us alone, our ears pounding with blood. I take Roni's hand and squeeze it, hard, because I can feel her slipping down the panicky slope.

"Listen—the babies are going to be all right," I say.

"Are you sure?" Roni says. Her eyes are red-rimmed with fear.

"Absolutely sure," I say, leaning in to her, my face set like stone. I am channeling Charlton Heston and Gregory Peck, so she cannot question my resolve. This is wishful thinking as much as anything else, but my mind will not accept the logic of climbing over so many hurdles only to be kicked to the ground now. Even if one of the babies has Down's syndrome, he or she will still be our child, and we will love him or her. So there is nothing for us to do except worry, and worry will not accomplish anything. The only option is to plow forward, as before, with hope and stale ginger ale and reruns of *Murder, She Wrote*.

.   .   .

By December Roni can barely climb out of bed. Her face looks as if she has lost thirty-five pounds. She is rail thin except for the fifty inches of mass that is her stomach. She literally looks wider than she is tall.

Her muscles are so weak from bed rest and her stomach so voluminous that she uses an old-lady walker to go to the bathroom, a distance of about fifteen feet. The sight of her leaning on the walker and hobbling across the den causes me to burst out in nervous laughter.

"It's not funny—I'm a prisoner in my own body," Roni moans. "I'm being taken over."

I can barely bring myself to gaze at her naked body. Her stretch marks have applied for workmen's comp. Her belly button splays out like a postmodern bathtub appliqué. Her poor breasts—she is well endowed to begin with—are abandoned across the Nepalese summit of her surging belly. But her shoulder blades and collarbone and cheek-bones jut out worrisomely.

At night, when the babies are most active, perfectly formed elbows and knees press out against the walls of her stomach, which gyroscopes in two or three different directions at once. I put my hand on her belly and feel punches and karate kicks. Asher holds up headphones and we play music for the babies.

My mom turns white and almost faints when she sees Roni's stomach.

"Oh, my God!" says my mom, who drives up from Philly to find out just what the hell is going on up here. My updates have been a little vague for her taste, as though I were an untrustworthy teenager calling in from a cross-country tour.

"It's going to be okay," I tell my mom, with a hug for emphasis. She is more worried than she can say. Her side of the family is all semiprofessional worriers, and she is the champion of the family tree.

"How is she going to last another month?" my mother says. "I don't see how she can get any bigger."

"We're renting some space downtown," I say. "Near the Holland Tunnel."

"What if there's a problem with one of the babies?" my mom says.

"Does this mean you're finally going to stop worrying about me?" I say.

"How far are you from the hospital?" she says.

I don't want her to even think about the traffic in Central Park, so I distract her by giving her a book to read with Asher.

Roni's mother is down for the day, too, and we bring Roni a snack. Roni can only manage a few bites before she becomes bloated. "I don't see how four people can survive on crackers and cream cheese." Roni's mother says. The babies press on Roni's stomach, diaphragm and bladder and leave her feeling continuously full, out of breath, and overdue for a trip to the bathroom.

I have reduced visitors to a minimum. Roni's condition is so alarming that the panicky look on people's faces is just too karmically negative.

Good news arrives when Roni finds out she has been voted into partnership at her law firm. She may be the only lawyer in New York to make partner while imprisoned in bed rest with a multiples pregnancy.

We celebrate with flat ginger ale in wineglasses, and rice crackers coated with a tiny smear of Cambozola cheese.

"You deserve this," I say. "You've worked like a dog to get where you are. They're lucky to have you." Roni savors the moment with childlike elation and surprise. This is an odd feeling for her, because she is not the self-promoting type. She may be a bit of a bullshit artist in the middle of a heated debate, but she never indulges in self-aggrandizement or ego trips. Seeing her like this brings me back to when we first dated and the more I peeled back the layers of her personality, the more endearing she became.

We see Dr. Rivera again at thirty-two weeks. The news is mostly good. The babies look healthy and well developed. At thirty-two weeks, the linings of their lungs are nearly mature, so even if the babies deliver now under emergency conditions they will be able to breathe without respirators. This is a major hurdle in our small neonatal world.

The bad news is that Roni is having minor contractions. Dr. Rivera tells Roni to begin taking the anticontraction medication. If the contractions become stronger or more frequent, Roni will be hospitalized. Dr. Rivera prescribes a fetal heartbeat monitor for Roni to wear all day and night, just to make her even happier.

I pull Dr. Rivera aside as Roni is dressing.

"Should we admit her to the hospital?" I say.

Dr. Rivera knows Roni. "She'll complain about having to use a bed pan, she'll object to having bloods drawn three times a day, she won't be allowed to take a shower—forget it," Dr. Rivera says. "Not to mention all the time I will be on the phone with the hospital administrator."

I agree. Then Dr. Rivera drops the really, really bad

news. Dr. Rivera may not deliver the babies. The week they are due, she is scheduled to be off duty.

Dr. Rivera patiently explains that she has kept one of her partners up-to-date on Roni's history, and how he is a wonderful doctor and surgeon. We meet the doctor and he is nice and smart and experienced, but this curve ball unleashes all the panic I have been suppressing. Before I know what is happening, I offer Dr. Rivera a bribe to be available when Roni delivers.

Roni turns to me with shock. "Did you just offer Dr. Rivera a bribe!?"

Dr. Rivera excuses herself.

I am red in the face. "Just a little financial incentive?" I say.

"I can't believe you did that!" Roni says. "Are you insane?"

"*I can hire Barbra Streisand to sing at a party for a million dollars,*" I say, defensively. "Why can't we get the ob-gyn we want?"

Roni stares at me the way she stares at Asher when he is hiding a stolen candy in his hand.

"I'm really, really sorry," I say to Dr. Rivera, when she returns. She understands the panic but needs me to know she has a husband and two small children and cannot be on call seven days a week, fifty-two weeks a year.

"Bruce offered the ob-gyn a bribe!" Roni says later that night, over and over again. She yaks on the phone with her mom and her sister and her girlfriends for hours. At least she has something to distract her from the heartburn and insomnia. And she hasn't complained about her bladder once tonight. If only the rest of my public humiliations could prove so productive to my loved ones.

FOUR

A, B, and C

Roni is in the bathroom, taking a shower, doing whatever it is she does. I can't go in there. She is a stick figure with a planet in her middle, blotting her out. Her stomach is an eclipse.

Asher gives Rosetta a hard time this morning, which is unusual. He throws his shirt on the floor. "Daddy, you get me dressed!" Asher says.

We still don't know where we are going to live. I am off to Riverdale, in the Bronx, to tour prefab 1970s apartments with brown shag carpeting. My aunt Rita, my dad's sister—the two have barely spoken for forty years—lives in Riverdale.

"Come on, Asher, be the good boy that you are," says Rosetta. We are lucky to have Rosetta. She loves Asher and has common sense; everything else is gravy.

"No, I'm a bad boy! Did you hear my words?" Asher says.

I turn away because I am smiling and do not want to reinforce this behavior or find myself in hot water. I am the easy one, Roni the disciplinarian. I overpraise, Roni is critical. On most questions of parenting, we are opposites.

My nature is to give Asher a small treat or two a day, to reward him, motivate him, or just to bask in that radiant glow of his two-and a half-year-old happiness.

But I battle my weight—as does Roni's mother—and she worries about Asher's long-term health. Left alone with him, she would permit a treat twice, or maybe three times, a week, to prevent him from connecting food with happiness and drowning his adult sorrows in cookies and ice cream and late nights at the McDonald's drive-through window. We bicker about treats, compromising somewhere around one treat every other day, with one extra treat on weekends. That puts Asher into the treat median, with many of his friends clocking in at two or three treats a day and a spare few with one treat a week.

In addition to my job as primary indulger, I am also the worrier-in-chief. When Asher has an earache, I rush off to the pediatrician, but Roni waits a day to see if he feels better. She does not want Asher to be afraid of pain, to be a weak and whiny adult, and she does not want to waste time and money on endless doctor's visits. She is concerned about the abuse of antibiotics, which, she has read, is creating new strains of supergerms. Our compromise is that Asher sees the doctor when he is uncomfortable and out of his element, but minor whining and complaining is treated as wait-and-see.

When Asher falls and skins his knee on the playground, I rush to his side, but Roni holds me back to let Asher pick himself up and evaluate the damage. If he is bleeding or wailing, I swoop in like an army ranger search-and-rescue team, but if he shrugs off the injury and returns to playing, so much the better.

When Asher misbehaves Roni insists on an immediate time-out, to which I agree, although I sometimes cheer him on silently because I want him to live life on his terms and not be a follower, even if it is our authority he is flouting. I want him to be well-behaved and obedient and polite, but I also want him to have a healthy sense of, as Groucho Marx said, "Whatever it is, I'm against it."

We argue about our dynamic constantly, but I suspect this is part of our attraction, that nature brings opposites together for reasons deep inside our DNA. When we are in a store and see a child misbehaving, his cowed parents powerless to stop the tantrum, we exchange a knowing glance. When hysterical moms rush to pick up their kids after a minor playground dustup, my skin crawls. When the waiter at the steakhouse leans over and tells us how impressive it is to see Asher sit so quietly during the whole meal, Roni turns to me for a hallelujah. We have been married five years now, and it is time to find a way to skip over the arguing and debating phase and jump right into the compromise. Roni agrees with this concept whole-heartedly. Then we argue about how to make it work.

Roni walks into the den, drying her hair. She leans over her walker like a tired old lady on the boardwalk in Atlantic City. We have made it to thirty-five and a half weeks. It is a Thursday. Roni's C-section is scheduled for next Tuesday. We have a long, relaxing weekend planned.

"I should be back by one-thirty. Do you want anything special for lunch today?" I say.

"Something different," Roni answers. She sits on the bed, combing her hair. I am happy to see she is feeling better, because she hardly slept last night, her stomach bubbling in protest. I ask what she means by different.

"I thought I'd have hospital food," Roni says.

"Why do you want hospital food?" I say, flipping through apartment listings.

"My water broke an hour ago," Roni says.

"What?" I say.

"Do you know where my blue sweater is?" Roni says.

I hear the words. I can see the words in the air circling my head, but they are not going in. I can feel the sweat coming, the adrenaline, my grinding and overheated glands.

"I don't . . . I don't . . ." I say.

"It's time, honey," Roni says.

"No," I say. "We're not ready. You're having your C-section on Tuesday." I look for the Planner where she writes down her daily schedule, to prove it can't be today.

"Get the bag, sweetie," Roni says. Rosetta squeals with laughter and sings and dances with Asher about the babies coming.

"But we have plans this weekend! It's not time," I say.

Roni calmly packs her bag while all the anxiety, fear, doubt, misgivings, insecurity, ignorance, and generalized free-floating negativity I have been holding back over the last eight months bursts out the top of my head like an ICBM breaking through its silo.

"Your water broke an hour ago?" I say. "And you took a shower?"

Roni is happy and peaceful. "I was all sweaty and yucky," she says. "I feel so much better now. Whew!"

"Mommy's having the babies, good job, Mommy!" Asher says, breaking in and giving her a hug. "Can I give them some candy for their birthday?"

My panic is aggravated by the smiley, oogly-googly good times swirling around me. "If your water broke, then the babies don't have anything to breathe! Oh, no!"

I am speaking loudly and walking around in circles. "We have to call Dr. Rivera! What's her number? What if she's not on call today! We need cash. Hooh! Ooooooo!"

"I'll call the mothers. Make sure you have the phone list," Rosetta says. She hands Roni her makeup kit, a hairbrush and a bottle of perfume, which, in the back of my overcrowded mind, makes no sense.

"Babies! Are the babies here? Babies! Come out come out wherever you are!" Asher sings at Roni's stomach.

"Okay! Okay! Okay! Let's just get organized!" I say.

I am not ready. I am not ready. I am not ready. What are the babies breathing if the water broke? I used to know the answer to this. I really am not ready.

"Are you all right?" the cab driver says.

We are in a yellow taxi rolling across Central Park and Ninety-sixth Street. It takes a minute to register that the cab driver is talking to me.

"Yes, thanks," I say. Roni looks out the window and smiles. It's a sunny, crystalline winter day. I am white as a sheet and sweaty and make small honking noises.

"Look at the flowers. Aren't the colors beautiful?" Roni says.

The cabbie is so busy watching us that he narrowly misses sideswiping a bike messenger, who screams and gives us the finger.

"What a beautiful day for a bike ride!" Roni says, rolling down her window.

Three hours later I am standing in a hallway on the eighth floor of the New York Hospital/Cornell Medical Center and pulling blue scrubs on over my clothes. The scrubs are tight—they only have XL, and I am XXL—and I sweat like a fiend. As I bend down to put on the soft blue booties, my head bonks a medical cart, rolling it down the hallway. A torrent of activity surrounds me—nurses, doctors, pediatric interns, anesthesiologists, and technicians. I feel an arm on my back.

"Don't worry, Dad," says a nurse, smiling through her surgical mask.

"Looking good," says a male technician, with a thumbs-up.

"Good," I say. I have no idea what I am saying. "Good. Mm-hm. Good."

I loop Roni's Nikon camera around my neck, where it dangles precipitously. I feel like an idiot. I am in near-cardiac panic, but I am ready to shoot some film!

Inside the OR, the activity level is intense, like a NASA control room right before liftoff. Every body, every object, every human motion has a distinct purpose.

Some thirty people are hard at work. A team of surgeons and assistants and obstetricians prep Roni. Three separate teams man three separate baby stations, each with a crash cart, EKG, and other emergency apparatus, and also the traditional warming carts, oxygen tanks, scales, footprint makers, Betadine, eyewash, suctioning tools. Each baby has a team of four to five people. Two or three anesthesiologists float around as Roni is gently transferred to the operating table and a green surgical tent erected over her midsection. Flat on her back she begins to gag.

"She has reflux—she can't lie flat on her back," I tell the nurses.

Roni's belly shimmies and shakes under the harsh lights. A nurse gently but efficiently scrubs down Roni's middle with Betadine.

"Hi, honey," I say. In addition to the epidural she has been hooked up to a Valium drip and is growing woozy.

"Make sure you watch them put the tags on their ankles," Roni says. After Asher was born Roni screamed at me, half-conscious, "Follow the baby!" Watching so much Lifetime TV has given her a switched-baby neurosis that has annoyingly enough wormed its way into my brain. I'm not sure how I will follow three babies simultaneously. I feel the weight on my neck—the camera. Must take pictures. Pictures.

The tempo in the room signals that surgery will begin soon, but I do not see Dr. Rivera. When I look down at Roni again, a small pillow has appeared under her head.

I hear the fetal heartbeats, see the bank of pulsing monitors. A surgical resident removes surgical tools from plastic sleeves and a sterilizer.

Dr. Rivera enters with an assistant, her face covered, her hair pulled back. I am always surprised by how small she is, given how powerful a figure she is in our lives. Dr. Rivera quietly begins giving orders.

"Everything looks good," Dr. Rivera tells me. With the mask on her face it almost feels as if she is communicating telepathically. "We're going to start. Just like last time, she's going to feel some pressure. Keep her calm, but let me know if there is a hot spot."

A hot spot is an anomaly—a portion of the body where the epidural is not working.

"Don't talk about me like I'm not—" Roni says.

I tell Dr. Rivera how wonderful it is that she happens

to be working today, how there isn't anyone else in the world that—

Dr. Rivera is gone. She is on the other side of the tent now.

I ask Roni if she wants the Walkman. I brought her favorite tape.

"Nat King Cole?" she says. I look down at the Drifters tape sitting in my hand.

"Go with the babies to the nursery," Roni says. "Make sure they do the—" She fades out for a blip.

"The footprints. Don't worry," I say.

"If anything happens to me—*ow!* I feel something!" Roni says.

Can they be cutting already? We just got here. "It's okay," I say. I don't know why I say this. A bomb might have gone off in Dr. Rivera's hands for all I know about what is going on.

"I feel that!" Roni says.

The nurse closest to me checks Roni's Valium drip. "I can't give her too much more," the nurse says.

"Shh," I say. "You're doing great."

"Don't shush me!" Roni says.

A nurse on the far side of Roni's stomach says, "Does it feel sharp, or do you just feel the pressure?"

"Knife," Roni says. "Knife!"

"We're dialed all the way up," the Valium nurse says.

"It's okay, honey," I say.

"Stop saying it's okay. That's always the last thing you hear," Roni says.

"All right, all right, now," I say. "Here we are now. Here we go."

Dr. Rivera's voice cuts through our conversation. "Roni,

I need you to take a deep breath now. Try to calm down, because we need to take the babies out."

Roni rocks backs and forth ridiculously on the table. I am confused. This is like a gag from the *Airplane!* movies. They shake her forward and back like a wax dummy.

The lights get hotter. I hear a ringing. White noise. Roni's body rocks up and back. She is now dozing, which seems ridiculous, given the level of chaos. I hear bells ringing, machines beeping. People move back and forth. My mask is wet with sweat and spit, slipping down my face.

A nurse says something. A heart rate dropping. Another nurse says something. Blood pressure. My head feels like a balloon that is being overinflated.

"Baby A is a boy," a nurse says.

The words seem very far away. What?

I look down at Roni. She is half-awake. I don't know if she heard this.

"A boy?" I say.

"What's wrong?" Roni says. "I don't hear anything!"

I look up and see Baby A being carried to the first baby station. He is swaddled in a white blanket, but he is quiet. A doctor suctions his nose and mouth, puts drops in his eyes, and listens for a heartbeat.

"Waaaagh!" Baby A says. His feet are pressed down for footprints.

Roni's body rocks up and back again. I worry she will sail clear off the table.

"Baby B, boy," another nurse says.

I see Baby B carried off in a different direction.

"Two boys!" I say to Roni. We didn't know what we were having. The ultrasounds were unclear on the sex.

I look at Baby A. There is a lot of activity at his station

now. I circle around to Baby B, who is crying a high, desperate cry. I see a stream of urine shoot into the air. Baby B is longer and thinner than Baby A.

Where is Baby C? Now there is a lull.

"Baby C is tucked underneath the internal organs. They have to be moved aside to get him out," a nurse says, reading my mind.

Roni's body rocks up and back again. More activity around Baby A.

"Baby C is clear. Baby C, a girl," a nurse says.

From somewhere back in the OR I hear clapping. I think. Clapping?

I ask the resident about Roni's condition. "She looks good," the resident says. "Give us a minute."

Baby C, the girl, is wailing loudly, a piercing foghorn of a scream. She has a thick head of black hair. All the babies are a good size. They are regular-looking babies, not preemies, with nice round heads, having avoided the crush of the birth canal. Now I remember what I have been trying to forget: The twenty-six-week ultrasound. The birth defects.

A nurse congratulates me. Baby A, she says, is five pounds and three ounces. Baby B, four pounds, five ounces. Baby C, four pounds, eight ounces.

"But are they okay?" I say. "Ten fingers, ten toes? You know?"

The nurse doesn't answer. She is looking at Baby A.

"Baby A has to go to NICU," she says. "He's having a problem we call grunting."

" 'Grunting'?" I say. Baby A is whisked out the doors inside an incubator.

"Baby A is breathing rapidly and his chest is compressing," says one of the pediatric interns. "We need to make sure he hasn't aspirated any amniotic fluids, or is having some sort of respiratory problem."

"But he's healthy?" I say.

"We'll know more in a few minutes," the intern says. "We're taking him to the fourth-floor neonatal ICU. Follow us down in about ten minutes."

"I have to go check up on Baby A," I tell Roni. "I'll be back in a few minutes."

Roni grips my wrist, stopping me from leaving. For a woman who is five feet tall, Roni is strong as a horse. She is rolling around in the Valium bog.

"Me dizit," she says, with tears in her eyes.

I think about that for a second. "No," I say. "*You* did it," I say, and kiss her on the forehead. Slimy globules of sweat drip down onto her face. "I'm really sorry about that," I say, wiping them off with my scrubs. "Can I have my arm back now?"

I sit outside the NICU unit. It is ten minutes later. My legs are like cement piles. Inside the NICU rows and rows of tiny babies are hooked up to big blinking machines. All that technology should make me feel better, but it makes me worry about the universe of complications babies face, their intense vulnerability. We hadn't even addressed the Down's syndrome question yet. They will have to run tests. There will be a period of not knowing.

I am mumbling to myself. A janitor—black, in his mid-thirties, wearing a Muslim head covering—asks if I am okay, if I need any help.

"No, thank you," I say.

He pushes his cleaning cart aside and sits down next to me.

"You got a baby in there?" he says.

"Yes," I say. "I mean, no. I have three."

He looks a little confused. "Three babies?"

"Yes," I say. "Triplets."

"Yeah, they get a lot of that here, because of the baby clinic. That is something, isn't it? Three babies! God must love you something special to bless you with three babies, mister. Let me shake your hand."

I take the janitor's hand and I start to cry, which is embarrassing enough in itself, but even more so thanks to the thick rope ladders of snot hanging off my face. The janitor gives me a paper towel from his cart. Incubators go in and out of the NICU, some with babies, some empty.

"Don't you worry—these doctors, they're gonna take good care of those babies of yours. God bless you, mister. You take care of yourself, now."

I thank the janitor, wipe my nose, and go into the NICU to see about Baby A.

"S-T-O-C-K-L-E-R," I say. I am saying it louder. They don't have my baby in here.

"Maybe they took him to the step-down unit," the receptionist says.

"No, I don't think—I don't know," I say.

Finally a nurse comes over. "Excuse me—your wife's maiden name?"

Then it hits me—*"Fischer."* The hospital always uses the wife's maiden name. When I donated my sperm they wrote *Fischer* on the specimen cup. Using the wife's maiden name eliminates one layer of confusion.

"Right!" I say. "Baby A, Fischer."

"The triplets. Congratulations, Mr. Fischer," the nurse says.

"Baby A has gone up to eight," says a supervisor. For a moment I panic. Gone up to eight?!

"That's the step-down unit," the supervisor says. "The three of them will have their own step-down unit, with their own nurses, around the clock. There will be a pair of twins in there, also, it looks like. Busy day today."

The grunting cleared up quickly. Just one of those things. Baby A's lungs are clear of fluid, no sign of jaundice, everything is fine. I ask about birth defects.

"I don't see anything on the chart, but you'll have to check with the geneticist on call," the supervisor says.

I feel thirty pounds lighter. The thumping in my head gives way to a kind of oozing warmth—we're going to be okay. As I start to run out of the NICU the supervisor says. "Mr. Fischer?"

"*Yes!*" I say.

"Try to stay calm. With three preemies, there are going to be any number of minor crises to work through."

As I run to the elevators my neck starts to hurt. I am still wearing Roni's camera. I look down and the film indicator says 32. I don't remember lifting the camera off my chest, but I shot almost a whole roll of film of the babies in the OR.

"The babies are sleeping in their cookers," Asher tells my mom, who drove up from Philadelphia with my dad. Divorced since 1978, they rarely occupy the same space.

My mom hugs Asher. "They look so small," she says,

with tears in her eyes. "It's okay, Mom," I say. "Look how big and healthy they are. We're doing great. Relax."

It is dinnertime now. The babies are in the eighth-floor step-down unit, a small private nursery that holds up to six babies. The babies lie in three incubators, pushed up to the thick Plexiglas windows. Traffic from the maternity ward streams along behind us.

"Lift me up!" Asher says.

Roni's mother, Gertrude, whom everyone calls Ima, the old-fashioned Hebrew name for "mom," stares at the babies through the Plexiglas.

"None of them looks like our side of the family," Ima says, in her German-accented English. "I wonder if they used the right eggs."

"I can't believe it," my mom says. "They're so small."

My dad stands in the back of the hallway chatting with Roni's dad, Peter, whom we call Abba, the traditional Hebrew word for "dad." Abba is white-haired, in his late sixties, very fit and trim, and also speaks with a pronounced German accent.

"I can't see faces," my dad tells Abba. My dad is about five feet tall and thin. He is in his early sixties, but looks twenty years younger and resembles Alan Arkin, except with bulgier eyes, thanks to heredity and thirty-nine years of glaucoma. My dad is one of those tense, impossibly complicated men, a dense and forbidding riddle whom the larger world showed little interest in solving. He is a professional hypochondriac and suffers from dozens of health problems, both real and imagined and impossible to separate. He is partially sighted from the glaucoma and walks with a telescoping cane. When I was a kid, he had asthma and was allergic to house dust and cats and dogs and pollen. He made our furniture in the basement of our house because the furniture sold in stores was all "cheap" and "crappy," but he never painted or varnished any of it. He was hyperactive and had at least one full-blown nervous breakdown. Most of my memories are of him screaming at my mom and yelling and crying and apologizing to us. After the divorce in 1978 he promptly lost his half of the money from the sale of our house in the stock market and moved into a small Philadelphia row house, living like a college student, sleeping on a cot balanced precariously on the milk crates that he used to store his acres of obscure photographic textbooks, tools, and holographic equipment. He had mysterious heart problems in 1988, the diagnosis of which was an enlarged heart, for which he takes medication, diets, and exercises. He says he almost died. As with most of my dad's life, there is no way to verify or refute this fact. He enjoys the air of mystery he has created for himself. And he has made an energetic effort to be a better grandfather than he was a father.

"I'll have to wait until they take the babies out of the incubator to get a closer look," my dad explains to Abba. "I have an infection, though, so I can't get too close. I could be contagious. My doctors can't even diagnose what I have—that's the way it goes! Philadelphia is a pretty backwater town. You can't even get a taxicab. They don't know where they're going. But I'm lucky to be here today. My cardiologist says I should have died in 1988. I said I wanted to live long enough to dance at my boys' weddings. I never thought I'd see a day like this. It's a miracle, isn't it? Did I tell you my ballroom dancing is keeping me alive? I can't wait until Asher is old enough to go dancing with me."

"You'll see them, don't worry," say Abba, who is dry as

wheat toast. "We'll take you in there and get you close enough so they can crap all over your head."

An attractive nurse walks by and my dad's head swivels after her like a security camera. My younger brother, Paul, claims he has seen my dad reading the CNBC stock market crawl from across a room. This has gone on since we were teenagers.

Roni's older sister, Ruth, stands with her three kids, ages eleven, nine, and eight. They live upstate, near Albany. "Let's live a little. Who wants Indian food?" Ruthie says to the kids. They wrinkle their noses. "Do they have McDonald's?" says Ben, the youngest.

A step-down nurse waves to me, and I bring in the grandmothers. We wash our hands and put on sterile masks. From the other side of the Plexiglas the faces stare in silently.

The babies have IVs stuck into their tiny hands, with a glucose drip. Baby A, the grunter, lies on his back. He is the heaviest at five pounds, three ounces. His face is round, his cheeks chubby, and he is completely bald. He reminds me of Curly from the Three Stooges.

Baby B is thinner and frailer. He has the faintest wisps of blond hair and is the smallest at four pounds, five ounces.

Baby C is the girl. She is four pounds, eight ounces, has dark hair and icy blue-gray eyes, but her most prominent feature is her uncanny resemblance to my dad. She has the same bulgy Stockler eyes I can trace back more than a hundred years from old family photographs.

"My God, she looks just like Len!" Ima says, meaning my dad.

"Isn't she beautiful?" one of the step-down nurses offers.

"It's like Roni wasn't even involved, except to carry the babies around like a truck," Ima says.

"Mom, what's the matter?" I say.

My mother is crying into a torn-up tissue. She is scared for the babies and for me and for Asher and the money and everything else, so I give her a big hug. Sometimes I worry that I am being condescending to my mom, because she worries so much, but her worry is purely out of love.

"This is why I'm so overprotective with Asher," I say. "Because of you."

"Asher should have on more than a T-shirt," my mom says. We both burst out laughing because she just can't help herself.

Ima points at Baby B. "This one, he doesn't look like anyone," Ima says.

In the hallway, Ben and Andy, Roni's nephews, take turns lifting Asher up to the glass. Abba reads *The New York Times*. My dad chats with a good-looking nurse, spreading the dedicated grandfather routine on nice and thick.

A step-down nurse lifts Baby A out of the incubator and puts him in my arms. It's confusing, because he is still attached to an IV and a heartbeat monitor, but he snuggles in. I take the tiny baby bottle and place it in his mouth, tickling his gums. It takes a while but he finally begins sucking.

"He look like your grandfather—look at the forehead," Ima says.

My mom is looking at Baby C, the girl. She must be horrified by the resemblance to my dad. It dawns on me that when Roni breast-feeds our daughter she will find her father-in-law's face staring back at her. This is a Freudian maze I do not want to enter.

I sit with Asher in a waiting room while he eats a candy bar. The family is going back to our apartment to have dinner. Rosetta talks to my mom in the hallway, both women casting waves of protective warmth in Asher's direction.

"Listen, Asher," I say. "Daddy and Mommy have to stay at the hospital for a week or so to take care of the babies. You will come here and visit us every day, okay? And I'll come home to tuck you into bed every night, and read you a story. All right?"

"No, you come home with me, Daddy," Asher says. "Mommy will take care of the babies." He climbs into my lap and asks for another candy bar.

"Listen," I say. "With the new babies, and the diapers and bottles, it's going to be a little crazy around the house, but I want you to know something."

"Are the babies going to sleep in my bed?" Asher says.

"No," I say. "Listen. Whenever Daddy is busy changing diapers or washing laundry, and you want to play a game or something, if I'm busy, I'm going to go like this." I hold up my index finger and make a number-one sign.

"See, this means number one. Because you're my number one. And I love you so much. And that will never change. Do you understand?"

"Okay, if I'm a good boy then can I have a candy bar when I get home, but not before dinner, because if that's not counted as a treat can I have a cookie after dinner? When I get home?" Asher says.

"Did you hear what I said about being number one?" I say.

"Because cookies are treats except for muffins, right? Only candy you have in a bag is, but not if it's little, then it's not a treat, not candy, right, a little bit, Daddy? Only sometimes it is a treat in your hand, if it's big."

"Don't eat too much candy," I say. "Otherwise you'll get a belly like Daddy."

Asher leans back in my lap. "I love you, Daddy," he says. He puts his hand up to my face. "My daddy."

I wash Roni's face with a warm washcloth. The maternity ward is quiet. It is eleven o'clock, but the hour means nothing in the backwash of this weeklong day.

"One of the boys looks like me, the second boy is a mystery, the girl looks like my dad," I say.

"I don't think so," Roni says. She looks strange and alien—thin and pale, suddenly fifty pounds lighter, crumpled up inside her own skin.

The girl is down in the NICU because she has reflux and is not keeping her formula down, so a feeding tube now snakes into her stomach. Also, she has mild jaundice and must go under the lights. Baby B, the thin one, also has mild jaundice, and also went down to the NICU under the lights. But no sign of birth defects so far.

"We're lucky," I say. We ignored the complications, the risk factors, everything. "There was another set of triplets born today," I say. "All under two pounds. They're all in the NICU."

"We're lucky," Roni agrees.

It's time to name the babies, I say.

"Can't we do it tomorrow?" Roni says.

Not a chance. When Asher was born, we couldn't agree on a name. For months before Asher was born we argued up and back, with zero agreement. I preferred Biblical names like Ezekiel and Zebadiah, and Roni wanted earth names like River and Wind and Tree. We couldn't have been further apart. We didn't name Asher the day he was born, or the following week, and the stalemate carried straight into the eighth day, the day of circumcision, which is also the day the baby is given its Hebrew name. For eights days our moms would call and ask, with great sarcasm, "How's *what's-his-name* doing?"

This time we have a girl's name picked out—Hannah—after Roni's grandmother, Aranka. We both like Jared. That leaves the second boy's name in dispute.

Roni likes Zane, Jordan, and Zoltan. I like Barak, Ezekiel, and Zacharia. I write the six names down on scraps of paper and drop them in an unused bedpan.

"You've got to be kidding," Roni says.

"If we don't do it now, he'll never have his name," I say. "And we still have to pick out the middle names."

Each of our kids will have one earth middle name and one family middle name. They will have five names altogether, like Asher, who was born within ten seconds of midnight and has Midnight as one of his middle names. Somewhere.

I swish the papers around and Roni picks.

"Barak," she reads. This is a mildly obscure Hebrew name that translates as "lightning."

"Two out of three," Roni says.

I toss the names in the garbage. "No, it will never end. You'll want to do a thousand and one out of two thousand. Forget it. It's Barak. Barak Stockler."

"They'll call him Rocky," Roni says. "We'll have to buy him the hat with the ear holes cut out." I know Roni means the gloves with the fingers cut off. Roni doesn't care about pop culture, and I have to translate her Norm Crosby-ish malapropisms about modern life into normal conversation.

"When are we going to Italy?" Roni says. I'd promised that if she was a good girl, stayed in bed, and made it to thirty-six weeks, we would spend two weeks in Tuscany.

"But you only made it thirty-five and a half weeks," I say. "Sorry."

"Go buy an Italian guidebook and check up on Jared, Hannah, and Zane," Roni says.

Roni and I both happen to be staring down at the blanket where her stomach is covered, and the sight of her normal-looking body now strikes us both as bizarre and miraculous, and we both burst out laughing. I gently rub her belly for good luck.

The quiet of the maternity ward is eerie. I have that disoriented feeling you get after body surfing in rough ocean too long. Clutched in my hand is the crumpled-up phone list. I don't have the energy to make any more phone calls.

I go down to the NICU and tell Baby B his name is Barak. He is sleeping quietly and has plastic lids over his eyes to protect him from the jaundice lights. I tell Baby C her name is Hannah. She has the covers over her eyes too and a small tube snakes into her mouth and down to her stomach, which makes me gag.

There are seventy-five or eighty babies in the NICU. Some only weigh a pound and are hooked up to a dozen devices. The nurses and doctors share a gritty trench-warfare confidence and the NICU hums with an electric intensity of purpose. But I can't look at sick children without feeling overwhelmed. I want my babies out of here.

Up in the step-down unit I tell Baby A, my big boy, his name is Jared. I watch Jared being fed and my peace of mind vanishes. The nurses feed newborns in an awkward position, sitting the baby upright, leaning them forward, and cupping the baby's chin in their hand. It's not a natural position but reduces reflux. I don't like how the nurse is handling Jared, though. She seems rough.

"Hey, how about if I feed my guy there," I interrupt. The step-down-unit rule is that you can handle your baby anytime except during rounds by the pediatric chief resident. The nurse hands me Jared. I take the bottle, lay him in my left arm, snuggle him in, and feed him. The nurse shoots me a look. I smile back. She is fucking with the wrong diaper jockey.

About twenty minutes later Dr. Drinan, the chief pediatric resident, enters with his interns and residents. Dr. Drinan says Baby B (Barak) should be out of the NICU tomorrow—his bilirubin count is almost normal. Baby C (Hannah) will not be discharged from the unit until she holds down at least six straight feedings. It might be four or five days.

Baby A, Jared, has hydronephrosis, an enlarged right kidney, consistent with what the twenty-six-week ultrasound showed in utero.

I am confused. I thought the enlarged kidney was a marker for possible genetic problems, not an actual physical problem itself.

"An enlarged kidney will often resolve itself in utero,"

Dr. Drinan says. "But the latest ultrasound shows what may be a pinch in the ureter coming off the right kidney. If the ureter is constricted, that could be preventing the kidney from emptying properly, and we'll have to keep an eye on it."

"What do we do if the kidney doesn't shrink?" I say.

"We'll wait a while, but if there's no change, or the enlargement grows, we'd need to do corrective surgery," Dr. Drinan says.

The doctor, despite the fact that he looks like a silver-haired alpha male straight out of central casting, sees the whites of panic cross my face. He puts his perfectly manicured hand on my shoulder.

"We're extremely conservative in cases like this," Dr. Drinan says. "No one wants to operate on a newborn unless it's an emergency. Most cases of this type resolve themselves naturally in a month or two. In fact, the improvement in ultrasound technology raises the question of whether we are prematurely diagnosing problems that naturally resolve, and creating unnecessary anxiety for the parents. But now we can identify and fix problems before they become life-threatening."

"So this blockage. It's like a straw that gets pinched shut? And you think it may have already unpinched itself?" I say.

"That's what we hope. We'll do a weekly ultrasound, then review in two months," Dr. Drinan says. He congratulates me and leaves with his team.

A nurse is diapering Jared. The diaper is too tight for my taste; they favor a clean incubator over an aerated rear end.

"Why don't you go get some sleep, Mr. Fischer?" the first nurse says.

"Yes," says the second nurse. "You won't be getting too much sleep for a while. Get it while it's good."

I'll leave in a minute, I tell them. "How about if I take care of the diaper first? I need the practice."

FIVE

The Wife We Never Had

I call my friend Rose Caruso to say hello. "Hello?" says her husband, Alan.

"Hi!" I say. "It's Bruce. Is Ro around?"

"No," Alan says. "She's sleeping."

"We had the triplets!" I say. "What the heck is going on down there in Montclair, New Jersey, with the whole sleeping thing when your friend is calling with triplets!"

"Bruce," Alan says, patiently. "You called us this morning."

"You did?" I say.

"It's four o'clock in the morning," Alan says.

"I don't know what time it is!" I say. "It's much colder in the hallway!"

"You need some sleep," Alan says, with his doughy Mel Brooks delivery. "But, hey—thanks for the wake-up call."

It is now the end of the triplets' first day, or the second day, depending on how you are counting. The babies were born after 2:00 P.M. on Thursday, but by the time everything calmed down it was one or two in the morning Friday, so I think of today, Friday, as the first day, even though this is technically wrong. Well, it's late Friday night or early Saturday morning now. That much I know.

Roni pumps breast milk and sleeps. She is ground up from the surgery and looks crazily thin. She lost fifty pounds of baby, placenta, amniotic fluid, and who knows what else, and looks strange and alien now. She is only half there.

Roni wants plastic surgery on her stomach. Plastic surgery, a trip to Italy—the costs are mounting and we haven't bought any diapers yet.

Barak has now joined Jared in the step-down unit. Hannah is still on the feeding tube and is not gaining weight.

I bounce between Roni, the step-down unit, the NICU, and our apartment like a sweaty bolt of lightning. The moms and the circles of friends require constant updates. Lawyers from Roni's office drop by to visit, which I find intrusive and voyeuristic, almost hostile, considering her frayed condition. My friends will not visit for a week, until Roni is back on her feet.

I make frequent stops at take-out joints for Roni, who endured thirteen or fourteen weeks without one enjoyable meal. Her heartburn and reflux are suddenly resolved and her internal organs have settled down after the Mardi Gras of the C-section, so she craves a dozen meals, some old, some new—eggplant parm, spicy Brazilian chicken, lean pastrami on rye, Milano cookies, babaganoush with pepper crackers, gorgonzola cheese.

.   .   .

At about 1:00 A.M. Sunday night I snooze on the floor on the mattress I removed from the rollaway cot. I can sleep until Jared and Barak are brought in for the 6:00 A.M. feeding, but I want to get up for the 3:00 A.M. feeding because I am still suspicious of the way the step-down nurses feed the babies. We are bumping along in a leaky raft on our never-ending day. My mind itches as if I have forgotten something important. Is Asher safely in bed? Will three baby seats fit in the back of a car, or will we need a van? Where are the babies going to sleep? Are we getting a baby nurse? If Roni goes back to work in two or three weeks, who's staying home with the babies? Can I get coffee now? Is that a bug on my leg?

Because of Roni's slow recovery, the hospital allows us to remain in the maternity ward for seven days. We worry about Jared's enlarged kidney, but it is not the health issues, caring for the babies, juggling work, or lack of sleep that stress us out. Our problem is disorganization. We're not ready for this. We don't have systems up and running, a master plan drafted, a road map laid out. We don't even have diapers yet.

Most married couples are like two pieces of a jigsaw puzzle, their strengths and weaknesses fitting together, however oddly the edges match, to make a whole. One is clean, one is sloppy. One shops, one cooks. One does breakfast, one does dinner. One partner covers the other's shortcomings.

But we are slightly out of balance as a team. We are both disorganized. We both pay bills late, forget to return phone calls, lose wedding invitations, order the wrong spare parts, leave the package on the supermarket counter, forget to turn off the lights, mix up play dates, leave the laundry in the basement after closing time, forget people's names who we see all the time, lose vital phone numbers, let birthdays slide away unacknowledged.

We are trying to divide and conquer our deficiencies before they do the same to us. I take over most of the bills, the laundry, the groceries, all the grunt work, which I don't mind. Roni is in charge of returning phone calls, play dates, birthdays and dinner parties and weddings. Shopping for the house and the kids is still our greatest failure, but, so far, Roni seems to be better at buying and I show promise in the returning.

But we are barely treading water, even working together. We are unprepared to organize the project of caring for three newborns and a three-year-old. We possess the love, the time, the commitment, the brains, the work ethic and, we hope, the energy. What we really need is a wife.

So Roni goes out and finds one.

Her name is Myrtle, a newborn-baby nurse who specializes in multiples. When Myrtle walks into the apartment, everything changes. Myrtle is General Patton in nurses' whites.

Myrtle is in her late forties, about five feet four inches tall, heavyset, with strong arms and legs from years of labor. She is from Trinidad and Tobago and speaks with an island accent that becomes thicker whenever she is critical or sarcastic. Her booming voice resonates with laughter.

When Myrtle arrives I am in the kitchen, boiling nipples, rinsing baby bottles, putting bottle caps on a drainer. Water is spilled across the tile floor of the unfinished tile floor. The sink is full of grimy dishes. The electric bill is floating in a two-quart saucepan full of oily water. The half-stripped kitchen cabinet doors lie propped up against the half-stripped counter, as they have for five years.

Myrtle begins bossing Roni and me around with her coat still in hand. This is fine with me, because we are unprepared for having the babies home. Myrtle looks around the apartment disapprovingly. She pulls out one of the red hospital-issue nipples foundering in the boiling water.

"Go throw these nipples out and get me some regular, old-fashioned, milk-drinking nipples," Myrtle says. She stares at me, unblinking. Myrtle means now. As I head for the door of the apartment, I turn back to see Roni smiling.

"What is this?" comes Myrtle's voice, from the kitchen. "No, no, no!" The smile disappears from Roni's face. Let's see how she handles the state of being perpetually wrong—that is, to feel like a husband.

Myrtle has long, flowing red hair, like a country-western singer. I notice it the first day, but in the craziness of our adjustment think nothing more of it.

On the second day, however, Myrtle's hair is piled up in a towering dusky orange beehive. Being bald and naturally indifferent to hair issues it takes me another day or so to realize Myrtle is wearing a succession of wigs, each more outrageous than the last.

"Of course she's wearing a wig!" Roni says, laughing at my ignorance. Women know about hair issues the way men know box scores. Unfortunately, I know nothing about box scores *or* wigs. I thought wigs were used in the movies. Women actually walk around with wigs on? This is news to me. Is it glued on?

"Every day is different, so why not look the part?" Myrtle says, when I work up the nerve to ask her. "Plus, it saves me a lot of time washing my hair. I just take me a new head out of the trunk and I'm ready to go." I stare at Myrtle's hair. Myrtle is like a performance artist, except she only performs to please herself.

The phone rings at 11:00 P.M. One of Roni's deals hit a snag with the SEC and she must do research for an 8:00 A.M. conference call. We have been home from the hospital three nights now and I am angry. Roni tells me to chill out, and stays up until 4:00 A.M., then spends half the next day straightening out the matter. Roni has always worked brutally long hours and I don't know what is worse, the shame I feel during those rare outbursts when she complains I should support the family, or the anger I feel at the roughness of her workdays. Oddly enough, my film magazine and her law firm—two businesses that couldn't be more different—share the same problems of mismanaging employee morale.

It took two maternity ward nurses about twenty-five to thirty minutes to feed the three babies a two-ounce bottle of milk. Myrtle quickly rinses the new nipples in boiling water, widens the nipple hole with a pin—"The babies want to eat, not blow up a balloon"—and sits down on our bed with the three babies splayed across her lap.

Myrtle puts two babies on either side of her right thigh, like two people lying down head-to-head at the beach. The third baby rests on her left thigh. She holds two bottles of milk in her right hand, facing in opposite directions, and feeds the two babies at the same time. She picks up the third bottle in her left hand and feeds the third baby. She starts singing an island song and examines *The National Enquirer* spread out around her.

Roni and I stare at each other. We have seen a lot, but it never even occurred to us two or more babies could be fed at the same time.

"Takes some practice, but you'll get the hang of it," Myrtle says.

Roni and I stand around, dumbstruck. "Why don't you go in the other room and sit down," Myrtle says. "I'll make you two some dinner." Then she laughs her Myrtle laugh, a heaving ho-ho-ho with her ample grandmother's bosom shaking up and down.

Roni and I check on Asher, sleeping in his Fisher-Price car bed in the living room. We sit in the den, still organized for Roni's bed rest, her walker propped up in a corner. I see empty cracker boxes and used-up cream cheese containers and seltzer bottles stuffed in nooks and crannies of the room.

"She can't burp them three at a time," I say. "It's not possible."

"Did she say she was going to make *dinner*?" Roni says.

"She was just kidding," I say. "Right?"

We look at our to-do list, longer than a Dead Sea scroll. I have to see a house in Bronxville, a small town at the southern tip of Westchester County. We want to move out of the city by March 1, now just three weeks away. We must find a house or apartment, sublease our apartment, and pack it all up—no small task, since it is as crammed full of junk as an old curio shop. We need a mover. We need to buy a car, a truck, an SUV—a vehicle to hold seven. We need a warehouse store that sells diapers and formula and other items yet to be itemized and budgeted. Baby gifts must be sorted and the critical items extracted— onesies, a diaper pail, baby blankets. We need two more cribs.

"Let's just sit," Roni says, when I read the list with increasing disbelief.

"But—" I say.

Roni takes my hand and pulls. I sit down. She's right. We should listen to our wife.

An hour later we are eating in our eat-in kitchen, which, in six years, we have eaten in exactly twice. We are eating home-cooked fried chicken, turnip greens, and the best sweet potato pie—the best pie—I ever tasted.

The kitchen is spotless. It hasn't been this clean since before Roni moved in.

"Do you think there's heavy cream in the pie?" I say.

"Does it matter?" Roni says.

The babies sleep quietly on our bed, fed and burped. Myrtle has created a barrier on one side of the bed. She lays the babies down in a row and climbs in and forms the other barrier. The babies are safe and sound, with nowhere to go. . . .

On their stomachs!

Like a slap in the face, I realize Myrtle has put the babies down on their stomachs. I didn't notice before, because she usurped our bedroom and we had to improvise.

I frantically motion to Roni about the babies being on their stomachs, but she fails to understand my sign language for two unforgivable minutes. Finally, it clicks, and

I see her face fall. We fight that teapot whistle of hysteria sounding in our brains.

"Uh, Myrtle, we uh—" I stutter.

"—Ah!" Myrtle says, holding up a beefy hand against my panicky face.

"Honey, now you're going to tell me all about them doctors and their back sleeping and their side sleeping and all that nonsense," she says in her lilting voice. "But I'm here to tell you that babies like to sleep on their tummies, and it keeps them from choking on their own spit-up just fine, and that's how it's gonna be. You'll see." Myrtle chortles quietly to herself, as though the fumbling ignorance of college-educated parents proves her most reliable source of entertainment.

Roni takes a big bite of sweet potato pie. Maybe the pie is a trick, I think—to make us sleepy and defenseless.

"I'll make up the bed in the den," I say, retreating.

"That's a good project," Myrtle says after me.

As I flee, Myrtle says to Roni, "Why don't you go have him give you a nice big foot massage, honey? And tell him to keep going until he finds a soft spot. Ah-haaah!"

Myrtle sits on the bed, the triplets arranged around her, the goddess of baby island. She reads *The Star* and *The Enquirer* and laughs out loud at the stories, her firecracker red hair shaking as it cascades down her back.

I haul Asher's old crib up from the basement storage room. We thought the babies could sleep three in a row in one crib until they are two or three months old. Multiples are supposed to sleep together.

"Get rid of this," Myrtle says. Myrtle pulls the sliding gate up and down and makes it squeak dramatically. "No good. You can't be reaching in and out of this thing all night long. Your back will be breaking in half."

Roni and I look at each other. Three or four times a day we find ourselves staring at each other as our opinions sink under the sandstorm of Myrtle's authority. Where are the babies going to sleep all night? In bed with Myrtle?

Myrtle climbs into our bed. The babies are safe and secure. She rubs them gently on their backs. In a few minutes she is snoring like a jackhammer.

Myrtle allows us to sleep through the night, an unimaginable luxury. Of course, for the first few nights I wake up, anxious and paranoid, at 2:00 or 3:00 A.M. I tiptoe down the hallway and pretend to use the bathroom, to spy on Myrtle, see if she is really feeding the babies or just sleeping through the night and faking it.

"Hello!" Myrtle sings, the first time my footsteps sound in the hallway. "You checking up on me, or do you have girly bladder? Huh-ha-hooooooo!"

"Both," I say. I leave the door open, so she can hear that I am indeed urinating.

"Hey, little dude," I whisper, pretending to adjust Asher's bedcovers.

"Go back to sleep, and stop worrying," Myrtle says when I peek into the bedroom. "Worrying don't do nothing but make doctors more rich." Myrtle gives me a big laugh and hands me a baby to diaper.

My dignity is restored, however, as she watches me, suspiciously, wondering how a man can diaper a baby so flawlessly. I feel so much better. It's always nice to show off for your wife.

. . .

At $2,100 a week, Myrtle earns nearly double my own salary, although she works twenty hours a day for seven days. My brother and, most surprisingly, the colleagues at my wife's law firm, each give us a week of Myrtle as an extravagant baby present. In the end, we have enough money for five weeks. Roni and I debate bitterly about spending so much money—but we are faced with such chaos that we give up and enjoy the luxury.

What makes this gift doubly special is that we can spend extra time with Asher. Asher is extremely curious about the babies and likes to pat them on the back to see if they will burp.

"They don't do anything," Asher complains.

On a warm day after work I take Asher to Riverside Park and tell him we are moving out of the city to live in a house. I am worried about how he will react. Like me, he is naturally cautious, loves routines, and sticks to the familiar.

"Can I have my own room?" Asher says.

I don't know what to say. Has he wanted his room all along? Does he understand that much about houses and apartments, or is he just fishing?

"If we rent a house, you can probably have your own room, but we'll have to see," I say.

"The babies cry all the time," Asher says. "I can't sleep in their room."

On the way home, we get pizza and stop in the bookstore, and as I look down our block toward the Hudson River and the lights of New Jersey, I feel a twinge of premature nostalgia. I am afraid of change. But if my three-year-old can get excited about moving, I should, too.

. . .

Roni spends considerable time pumping breast milk. She pumped for Asher until he was six months old and is determined to pump enough milk for each baby to have four or six ounces a day.

The breast milk pump is the most embarrassing contraption imaginable. It turns grown women into dairy cows, and the noise—*thwock-THWOCK, thwok-THWOCK*—is horrifying, like something from a Terry Gilliam movie.

"I don't understand why that makes you so tired," I say, as Roni sits, propped up in bed, grimacing. *Thwock-THWOCK!*

"Try putting your penis in a vacuum cleaner for half an hour," she says.

The milk is dribbling out. Roni barely generates six ounces at a sitting. I give Roni a drink and a snack and check in on the babies.

Myrtle's feeding of all three babies is a mystery of ergonomics I cannot decode. The babies are so much smaller than Asher that I cannot get comfortable feeding more than one at a time. And they eat much more slowly than Asher did, unless this is a trick of my memory. Am I thinking of him as a baby or as a nine-month-old, emptying bottles in the blink of an eye?

Myrtle regards the breast milk with skepticism. She has lined up a dozen full bottles. Everything is in order. She sees me fumbling to divide the breast milk evenly.

"Either it comes out or it don't," she says, shaking her short blue hair. "There's no sense torturing herself for this little itty bit of milk." I am not about to cite articles on the benefits of breast milk. You don't cite articles to a force of nature.

. . .

Myrtle feeds the babies, diapers, launders, washes, cleans, and cooks outrageous meals for us—ribs, chicken, dirty rice, collard greens, and that sweet potato pie—without breaking a sweat. She takes catnaps—fifteen minutes here, thirty minutes there—after the babies have eaten, day and night, so I never know whether she will be out cold and snoring or wide awake, waiting in ambush.

Myrtle loves trying to embarrass me. When she changes a diaper, she says, "Don't get no baby shit under your fingernails, cause it never comes out." When I bump into her in the morning as we juggle the bathroom, she says, "Gotta attend to my three *S*'s—shit, shower, and shave!" Myrtle says little about her personal life. She is who she is.

One day I come home from work to an amazing sight: baby Jared sitting in the kitchen sink. Jared is getting a bath in a small plastic tub as Myrtle cradles him in her hand and rinses him with the faucet. He squirms but does not cry, his chubby, bald head shining from baby soap. I haven't even considered giving them a bath yet.

One by one Myrtle takes the babies, washes them in the sink, dries them, diapers them, and wraps them in a thick, fluffy towel. I hold Asher up to see this amazing sight.

"Do they like it?" Asher says.

"I'm not sure," I say.

Myrtle makes possible the brutal job of boxing up our junk and moving it into the old, rambling house we rent. We have so much old junk shoe-horned into our apartment that I make eighteen separate runs to Bronxville in a rented step-van just to clear a path for the movers to extract our belongings. Eighteen trips and one hundred and fifty boxes just to make room for the movers.

On moving day, we leave the babies with David, Roni's boss and senior partner, Jodi, his wife, and their three girls. Nearly blocking West 114th Street, the twenty-foot moving truck is so crammed the movers warn us we will need a twenty-four-foot truck, a full tractor-trailer, next time. They can't believe how much stuff could emerge from a seven hundred-square-foot apartment. The chief moving guy (the most dangerous-looking one) says we are one of the few customers whose estimates have been wildly botched on the low side.

My mom works for GMAC and helps me with the paperwork on a Chevy Suburban, our first car, although we only get a 5 percent discount instead of the standard 15 percent, because the Suburban is so popular.

We enroll Asher, three now, in a little yellow schoolhouse around the corner from our new home on one of Bronxville's two main streets. The house is a 1920s Dutch Colonial in advanced disrepair. We put new carpet down in Asher's and the babies' rooms and paint all the upstairs bedrooms, but that is as much prep work as we can finish.

Asher gets his first big-boy bed, an antique mahogany twin bed Roni finds at a tag sale ($35). We erect metal shelving in his room and display all his toys for the first time. It feels therapeutic to crush and recycle some of the moving boxes that have been following us around and multiplying over the years.

Friends donate two cribs and we line the walls of the nursery with three cribs and the day bed. The room is sunny and warm and open.

Neither Roni nor I have lived in a house in twenty years. The first night we stare at the living room and dining rooms—actual, separate rooms. For years our rooms have been hyphenates—den-TV room-office-bedroom—but now the rooms have only one job each.

"A dining room table," Roni says, wistfully, her eyes scanning the empty, dining-tableless room. We hold hands and stand in the middle of the room. "Helloooo," I say, trying for the echo effect.

"I'm going to build a dining room table," Roni says. She walks off careful carpenter's footsteps. I find a hidden closet that will hold most of our china and serving plates, which means another ten or twelve boxes down.

And so it comes to pass that Myrtle must leave us after the five busiest weeks in our lives. We must buckle down and survive by our wits. We hear that Myrtle is off to work for Edgar Bronfman Jr., which confirms my suspicion that we are living far beyond our means.

Myrtle's husband loads her suitcases in the car and waits with the engine running. He doesn't say a word the entire time. I can only guess how shell-shocked Roni and I look, because Myrtle starts laughing at us. She gives us each a big, reassuring hug and a buss on the cheek.

"How much would it cost?" I blurt out. "Give me a number."

Roni looks at me, horrified. Here we go again.

Myrtle laughs at my suggestion. She enjoys the freedom of hopping from job to job, family to family, house to house. "You get to feeding them babies as good as you go diapering them, maybe I'll give *you* a job," Myrtle says, punching me on the back. Roni's eyebrow lifts up as she runs the numbers. Not to mention, it's a growth business.

Myrtle grips my arm. "Now, you sleep them on their tummies, like I showed you, make sure they get up a nice burp, rub their backs to settle them down, and, most of all, keep the radio on all the time, so they don't get to being sensitive to no noise," Myrtle says. "You don't want babies who wake up every time the wind blows or the phone rings or the dog barks."

Myrtle hands me two babies.

"Remember what I said about not getting baby shit under you fingernails, cause it never likes to come out! Haa-haaa-haaa!" she says, and sweeps out of the house, her bosom quaking with laughter.

For a brief moment the house is ghostly silent, like a church after the bells have stopped ringing. Then I hear Myrtle bossing her husband around outside, and then the sound of the Cadillac Deville gunning into the street.

I look down at baby Jared and baby Barak.

"Hi, guys!" I say. They begin to cry.

"I know, I know," I say. "I feel the same way."

Myrtle has bestowed upon me her meticulously maintained baby ledger. The baby ledger holds twenty-four-hour charts with separate line entries for each baby and feeding time. It records ounces of milk consumed, diaper contents, relative emotional state, hours of sleep.

I begin to freak out. Roni and I can barely pay the bills. But this baby diary is no joke. Hannah still has trouble keeping her food down. If Hannah's weight drops just one pound, she will be hospitalized in the NICU on a feeding tube again. One of us will have to stay over in the city, at the hospital . . . the logistics are impossible.

But it will be all too easy to forget the details at 3:00 or 4:00 A.M. when the babies are crying, diapers are flying, and we are trying to keep it all together.

"Put Post-it notes on their cribs, and change the color every feeding," Roni says.

"I don't know," I say, skeptical of my record-keeping abilities. "I just accidentally paid an AmEx bill from eight months ago."

The first night alone, Asher goes to bed in his own, brand-new bedroom after we read two Tom and Pippo books and watch the Winnie-the-Pooh video. The Winnie-the-Pooh video has been a constant from the time Asher was fifteen months old. I have seen the Winnie-the-Pooh tape literally five hundred times and can honestly say that I find something new in it every single viewing. (This makes *Pooh* and *Goodfellas* my two most-watched films of all time.) Although Asher is ready to graduate to another favorite tape, I coax him into watching it for my own comfort.

"Don't close my door," Asher says when I tuck him in. "I might need to tell you something important." I have no intention of closing his door.

"We're right across the hall," I say. I show him how close he is to our bedroom.

"Are the babies going to sleep in their cribs?" he asks.

"I hope so," I say.

Five minutes later I hear Asher saying "Daddy" in a low

voice, testing the security system. I cross the hall, sit on his bed, and reassure him we know what we're doing, even though we don't.

"I'm just checking," Asher says. I kiss him and tuck him in a little bit tighter. I know just how he feels.

SIX

I Sleep at Red Lights

The first night alone in our first house, the babies are just shy of six weeks old. When I peek into the darkened nursery, Roni is rocking a baby in the new leather-trimmed glider chair we bought after she rejected every one of the other 124 rocking chairs known to Western civilization.

"Look at my little stinky," Roni says, nuzzling Barak and giving him little pony bites. Barak is sleeping on the job again.

"Wake that boy up, or the whole system is going to collapse," I say.

It takes Roni an hour to finish the 8:00 P.M. feeding. I take Myrtle's baby book in the hallway and look at the numbers. My apelike printing makes my entries hard to understand next to Myrtle's flawless notations, neat as an Excel spreadsheet.

After Asher falls asleep we eat dinner in our bedroom. Every time we hear a moan, or a sigh, or a throat being cleared from the baby's room, we freeze.

"Noisy sleepers," Roni says. We debate keeping the babies' room door closed so that we only hear the most urgent crying, a kind of audio triage.

"What if someone is choking on their own vomit?" I say. "What if they are being strangled by the baby bunting?"

"Oh, God," Roni says, rolling over to look at me as if I am a chimp running around loose. We keep the door open.

My plan is to feed the babies at midnight, jump into bed, and sink into three hours of thick, oblivious sleep. Roni and I tentatively agreed that whoever woke up first would take the 3:00 A.M. feeding and the other person would handle the 6:00 A.M.

"What about in-between feedings?" I say. "The babies aren't going to wake up on schedule."

"Let's see what happens," she says.

"This isn't much of a system," I say, which is incorrect. In fact, our system has been carefully tweaked and patched together. Roni is the breadwinner, and I am the bread butterer. Roni is in charge, generally, and I am in charge of Asher. Roni works eighty to ninety hours a week in the office, I put forty in the office and forty or fifty at home. If Roni tends to hide under the covers when the screaming starts, how can I possibly object? If she is too tired to perform her job, we can't pay the rent, let alone the bills. Roni is the thin green line between us and a leaky one-bedroom apartment.

Roni has resumed her eighty-to-ninety-hour work schedule with just three weeks after the delivery to get back on her feet. The annoying night and weekend phone calls, the 8:00 A.M. Saturday FedEx deliveries, the condescending and nit-picking e-mails, the irrational clients—Roni's salary is practically choked out of her. One of the younger female lawyers sometimes steals into Roni's office to have a crying jag because of all the office stress. Roni is burned out after just one week back, but as a partner she is now expected to bring in business. In fact, as partner she is making less money, because she pays her own medical insurance, self-employment tax, and social security tax. So we are actually losing money unless she brings in new business, which means longer hours at conferences, networking, socializing—more stress and more hours away from home and the kids. Roni seems to be losing ground no matter how hard she runs.

It is you and me plus three, I tell Asher. Feeding the babies at night and changing their diapers and rocking them in the rocking chair will help me bond with them the way it did with Asher, I tell myself. Sure, I will have less time and energy for Asher, Roni, my job, the house, and myself, but careful planning will help me become a better family manager. I will become more efficient, more organized, more productive. If being father to Asher made me ten times the man emotionally, taking care of the triplets should expand my humanity 300 percent. As a mathematical ignoramus, this calculation is completely nonsensical, but it helps motivate me.

My goal is to try to feed two babies at a time, and then the last, the most finicky or pokey, completing one entire feeding in about forty-five minutes. If Myrtle can feed three at a time, then I can feed two. Diapers, another ten minutes—no man or woman alive is a more gifted diaperer.

Then I will try to catch maybe two and a half more hours of sleep before the 6:00 A.M. feeding. I can survive on that schedule, I say to myself. One day at a time now.

This is my plan, anyway.

Barak wakes up cranky at about 10:15 P.M. Barak has the saddest, most mournful cry. I walk him around on my shoulder for half an hour. He only needs twenty minutes to calm down, but ten minutes are for us to commune. Then Jared wakes up, unhappy. His cry is louder and insistent, more demanding. Jared is still awake at 11:30. It doesn't make sense to put him down now and wake him up again at midnight.

I decide to feed Jared and Hannah first, then Barak. But Jared needs to be held more than he needs to eat, and Hannah wants to sleep, not eat.

At six weeks, Jared is still bald, with just the slightest peach fuzz, round faced and chubby. He achieves the greatest total hours in crying but also quiets down the fastest once held. Jared is the least responsive to visual stimulus. He sits in the bouncy seat and stares off into space with a glazed, happy look. Roni's mother has started to worry that he is "slow."

By 12:30 I have fed, burped, and changed Jared and Hannah, but Barak, our sleepy fellow, is having trouble staying awake. I keep Barak on my shoulder and rub Hannah's back because she is gassy. I find myself slightly uncomfortable around Hannah and am at a loss to explain it. She is the only girl, and if this is the problem, I have no idea why.

It is just after 1:00 A.M. when I finish filling out the

baby book. I slide into bed, filled with pride. The babies are fed, clean, and sleeping soundly. If I can parachute into dreamland now, I will have two sweet hours of sleep before I hit the ground. The schedule is holding. Maybe this won't be such a—

A loud thump. I'm groggy, but the noise is a definite thump. I run through the scenarios—knock on the front door, falling pot, crappy old house collapsing . . .

No, no—I know what it is. I jump up and move quickly to Asher's room.

Asher kicked off his swaddling as an infant and never tolerated blankets. He has grown into a violent, gymnastic sleeper, gyrating across his bed in all directions. He rotates 360 degrees while he sleeps and some nights I find him upside down and hanging over the edge of his bed. When he visits the big bed he pistons Roni and me apart. Sometimes I wake from a falling dream to find Asher feverishly shoveling me toward the edge of my bed.

Asher is sleeping peacefully and comfortably on the floor, sucking on his two middle fingers, his rolled-up blanket intertwined with his body and his pillow resting on top of him.

I return Asher to his bed and arrange pillows on the floor to smooth any future landings. Since I am awake I double-check all the doors and windows in the house. The windows and doors are bothering me.

Most New York City apartments have only one door, leaving you sealed off from the outside world as if locked inside a bank vault. But this house has two doors and two dozen ground-floor windows that can be smashed or jimmied open. I haven't lived in a house since 1978 and had no idea how much New York City paranoia had poisoned my mind. I look at the cheap wooden doors and windows and think, *How do people live in houses?* Six-year-olds with Boy Scout knives could break into this house. But we live in a wealthy small town protected by a semifascist police force, so my city paranoia must be recalibrated to my suburban environment. As I walk by the front door, however, I realize we still have the same keys as the previous tenant. When I mention these problems to Roni, she calls me Mr. Security. Asher finds this hilarious. "Here comes Mr. Security," Asher says to his teacher when I pick him up at school.

Somewhere around 1:45 I climb into bed, close my eyes, and pull up the covers. My body slips instantly into a state of Zen-like tranquility, but as the cool comfort of the pillow ices down my aching head I hear crying. I fantasize that it comes from the house next door, where Roni says there is also a newborn. For another moment I imagine it is the TV. I look over at the alarm clock as it snaps over to 1:48.

Jared wants to be held again. By the time I extract him, his crying rouses Hannah, who wakes with ear-piercing screams. Her cries pulsate with anger and outrage.

I pace the second-floor landing in the dark, cradling the two caterwauling entities. As I march back and forth past Asher's room, I hear him talking in his sleep, which makes me wonder how he is handling the stress. Roni and I worked with him to prepare him for the changes, but I worry about whether this has helped. How can we prepare a three-year-old child for a transformation that threatens to overwhelm seventy-nine collective years' worth of parental intelligence? I freak out when the bagel store runs out of low-fat bran muffins, forcing me to eat the low-fat corn. Why should I expect Asher to show so much flexibility when I am such a spineless and pathetic creature of habit?

I walk with Jared and Hannah until about 2:30. I finally lay them down and get them settled when Barak cries out, cranky again, but still asleep. It takes a while to decipher what Barak needs—his Enigma code is the toughest to crack. I decide he needs another diaper, because his stomach seems upset, he has a slight case of diarrhea. I change him carefully. In the dead of night, the tearing of the Velcro sounds like a small woodland animal screaming.

I arrange the three babies on the daybed, as Myrtle did, then lie at their feet for a catnap. If I can cruise with them in sleepyland until 3:30, or maybe 4:00, I will be golden. The babies must be exhausted now. They need their sleep. They're babies, right?

Anyway, this is the plan.

Hannah wakes up eight or nine minutes later making a gargling sound. Reflux? I scoop her up and walk slowly, carefully, praying she won't spit up. She chortles and ha-hems and coughs and brings up clear phlegm, which eludes the baby blanket and trickles down my back, but she hangs in there and doesn't give me the Exorcist treatment. Good girl.

After a few minutes Hannah starts sawing happy little Z's. I put her down and adjust Barak, who now sleeps with his face straight down in the bed, nose crushed in on itself. Why do babies sleep nose-down in the bed? Are they purposely tormenting us? As soon as Barak is snuggled in he vomits explosively, all over himself, the bed, the blankets, the wall, and the floor. Waves of vomit surge in every direction.

I pick Barak up so he doesn't choke and the puke spills down my back and dribbles into my underwear.

"I don't understand," I say out loud. "Am I doing something wrong?"

Holding a tangle of vomit-drenched sheets, vomit dripping down my arms and legs and into the crack of my ass, I check in with Roni. "Honey?" I whisper, into the darkness. No response. I debate waking her, but she is exhausted. And my stupid male pride must be factored in. Waking her will be a moral failure.

"Marriage isn't a competition," a marriage therapist told us. Sure it is. Some men climb Mt. Everest, or sail across the Pacific Ocean in a bathtub, or run two-hundred-mile marathons. I will make it through tonight alone or die trying.

After a five-minute shower, my first break of the day, it takes about thirty minutes to decontaminate the babies' room as thoroughly as possible without tossing the mattress into a Dumpster. By then, Jared wakes up and wants to eat.

I feed Jared in the rocking chair, my back hurting from bending awkwardly over the daybed during the devomitizing. Then I feed Hannah and give Barak a bottle of Pedialite. I change all the diapers again and tie up the full diaper bag.

A full diaper pail is the nastiest stench in the world. I emptied Asher's diaper pail every twelve hours because I couldn't take the ripening tang. With the babies, I toss a bag out every six or eight hours, full or not. Sometimes, on a warm day, if the bag sits overnight, I feel woozy when the shock waves of odor blow up and scorch my face. I can barely imagine how much worse it will be once they hit solid food.

I carefully slide the diaper bag down the stairs, where it promptly breaks open. As diapers skid down the three steps and tumble into the kitchen, I pray the Velcro fastenings hold.

It is about 4:45 A.M. by the time the babies are sleeping. I lie down on the daybed because it is too painful to eject myself from the Hawaiian vacation of my own bed again. I hope to sleep until 6:00 or even 6:30. The babies must be tired from being up so much. Their little bodies need rest, sweet, rehabilitating sleep.

Isn't this a good plan?

I wake with a start at 7:30, sunlight inexplicably slicing across my eyes, my head and neck burning in pain. Rosetta is standing in the threshold to the nursery, laughing. I am slumped up against the radiator, Jared snoring in my lap. I barely remember doing the 6:00 A.M. feeding or how I ended up on the floor with Jared. I am disoriented, dream logic smeared over my face.

"Where's Larry?" I say. Rosetta laughs at me, takes Jared, and hands me her coffee to sip. Behind her Roni scoots down the hallway and into the bathroom, doing her kooky Lucy lateness routine with flying pantyhose and loose change spilling.

"Is everyone okay in there?" Roni says. "Oh, God, I'm so late!"

I go to the office feeling dipped in concrete. My arms and legs barely move and I crave a few hours in bed more feverishly than I ever craved sex or extra-cheese pizza. I am dismayed at my condition. In college I spent forty-eight or even sixty hours awake at a time. Now, of course, I am thirty-seven, and forty pounds heavier, which is a lot of years and too many low-fat bran muffins later. The 9:00 A.M. walk to the train station, just three-tenths of a mile, feels like a trek across an Arabian desert. I take the train to Grand Central, then the shuttle train to Times Square, then a local train south to Thirty-fourth Street.

I close my office door, too exhausted to chitchat, and focus on editing the stories for the current issue. Sometime after lunch I am startled to find I have been punched viciously in the forehead. When I come around, I realize I have dozed off at the computer, pitched forward, and slammed my head into the top of my Apple computer monitor.

I try slouching back in my seat, but that makes me even sleepier. The office maintenance guy turns off the heat in my office and cracks open the windows overlooking Eighth Avenue. I hope the cold will keep me awake.

On the way home, the subway trains are packed and the heat is on full blast. I hate the subways. My definition of wealth is never taking a New York City subway.

Grand Central is a human dodgeball game. Usually, I weave and bob and tuck through the teeming crowd like a college running back, without being touched, but today my rhythm is off and I am slamming into people left and right.

I dream of my childhood house, my baseball cards and my toys and my dog, Humphrey, running through my backyard with my little brother, when I am jolted awake by the sound of the word "Tuckahoe." Tuckahoe is the Metro North train station one stop after Bronxville. I slept right through my stop. Now I have to cross the tracks and wait for a southbound train.

The second night is remarkably similar. Myrtle's schedule will not work for me. The babies wake and need comforting, take luxurious amounts of time to feed, I hear or imagine noises, Asher talks in his sleep, I have an anxiety attack about a window or door left open. Roni sleeps soundly even after I poke her. Jared is gassy and fussy and I try sleeping with him lying on my chest, a blanket trussing him down to me to prevent him from falling, but I can't get comfortable enough to fall asleep. I worry I will roll over and crush him. He cries and wants to be walked around on my shoulder.

The weeks that follow pass in a blur of Tylenol and coffee and walking in circles in the darkness. At night I sleep in thirty-minute bursts, sometimes catching as much as an hour and fifteen minutes. I cannot fathom the scheduling mojo Myrtle conjured.

The Metro North train ride into the city provides one of my longest, uninterrupted sleeps of the day. I sit down with the *The New York Times* and by Fordham station in the Bronx I am out cold. This leaves fifteen to twenty minutes of cool snooze time before the train hits Grand Central, plus five more as the train empties. One morning I wake up to find myself alone on an empty train, the doors closed and locked, and I bang on the windows to draw the attention of a conductor.

Sometimes when I doze off I pitch forward and my head

rebounds off the Plexiglas train window. Sometimes my snoring shakes me back to reality and I look around, embarrassed, at the businessmen in their gray suits and pink faces. Sometimes I reflexively pull up out of a head bob so severely I threaten to crack a vertebrae. Then I start to laugh, because I know how ridiculous it looks to see a grown man perform a complete head bob and jerk awake, wet lipped with surprise. Snoring, head bob, laughing to myself—I should be pulled in for questioning any day now.

I sleep everywhere. In my office I balance a stack of press releases atop the computer monitor to block the view from the office floor, but when I doze off and head-butt the monitor, the stack of press releases and videotapes crashes to the floor and streams across my desk.

My office is small and everyone knows everyone's business. My co-workers pass by my office at an unusual rate, suspicious of my closed door, which I have always left open.

Sometimes I lean back in my chair, page layouts in hand, and doze off, waking with a panicky start as my chair threatens to pitch backward. Sometimes I struggle to remain conscious and frantically scribble on the layouts as Nicky walks by, pretending to get a drink of water or check the fax machine. He knows something is up. Nicky lives for sales projections and monthly quotas, and the unknown disturbs him. Nicky regularly jokes with the salesmen and clients how thankful he is to be divorced, how lucky he is not to have any rugrats hanging around his neck.

Nicky's attitude doesn't bother me. I don't feel morally superior to the childless. (I don't think I do, anyway. But who knows what darkness lies within the heart of a family man?) I am, unfortunately, the obvious odd man out at our parent company, which owns about two hundred magazines. I am the only dad with small kids in the New York office and I do not see the daddy track. The Midwest sales rep has kids, but he earns enough for his wife to stay home. Nicky's boss, the group publisher who is based in Kansas, has twins, but he earns a huge salary and his wife stays home to tend their McMansion. When I told Nicky it was unfair that the salesmen earned double or triple what the editors did, especially since they were selling our editorial reputation, Nicky laughed a big happy walrus laugh. "You get paid more the closer you are to the money," he said. I told him we should add that to the inspirational corporate posters (Innovation—Anyone Who Thinks the Sky Is the Limit Has Limited Imagination) sprinkled throughout the office.

One night Nicky sticks his head in my office while I am editing an assignment with Matt, the sharp twenty-something associate editor I recently hired. Nicky asks us to meet him for drinks at a hip midtown postproduction company that is completing some special effects for a big summer movie. Matt agrees and Nicky looks at me. I would love the break, but it would take at least a day to arrange a late night out. I tell Nicky I can't make it, but will schedule a visit to see the special effects. Nicky cracks a joke about how hard it is for women to juggle their priorities. When Nicky leaves I tell Matt that he might have my job someday, as long as he doesn't pop out any kids.

I have been avoiding the issue of my work life. In our little corner of the film world, my job carries a fair amount of clout—big fish, very small pond. Should I look for a similar job at a consumer magazine, like *Premiere* or *TV Guide*? Are there any editorial jobs that would even pay enough for Roni to stay home? My Achilles heel was in the networking. Like most industries, media jobs were based on connections, and I spent no time cultivating friends at consumer magazines. Instead, I spent the last twenty years hopelessly trying to sell my screenplays or get a staff job writing for David Letterman or SNL or Comedy Central. Maybe it was time to turn my creative energies into starting a business.

Tanks of coffee help in the morning but cause painful cramps and nausea by late afternoon. I switch to carbs for the glucose rush, but with my workout routine reduced to walking up and down the stairs for diapers and bottles, my pants are tightening like a noose. Shooting up another pants size will be a very negative complication now.

One night after dinner, I fall asleep on the toilet and wake up, suddenly, as my face slides down the tile wall with an abrasive screech.

"Daddy!" Asher says from the doorway. "What are you doing in here?"

Sleeping, son. Your father sleeps on toilets. Sometimes I take vacations in the sink.

I run through my backyard with my beagle, Humphrey. My brother, Paul, and I chase him around, make him fetch, and wrestle with him in the grass as he jumps all over us and paints us with hot doggie kisses. Woof! Arooo! I jerk rudely awake to the faces of subway riders staring at me. I am on the subway to Grand Central, sleeping, standing up, my hand gripping the overhead metal strap, an urban tree sloth.

I change my driving habits. When I run out for milk or diapers late at night, I put the car in park at red lights so I can lean my head back and snooze for a minute or two. If it is after midnight, I doze even longer, until I hear a car horn blast behind me. I pick the routes where the lights stay red the longest.

I sleep in elevators, leaning on the wall and going up and down a few extra times. I sleep in line at the bank and at the Mongolian barbecue restaurant across from my office, putting my head into my hand. I sleep in cabs the way people sleep after surgery.

Sleep deprivation is a classic technique of psychological torture. I grow snappish and irritable, but recognize this and try hard not to yell at poor Asher. This leaves Roni as the sole object of my foul moods, and she obliges my misdirected hostility by arguing back over the endless housekeeping details and, eventually, our division of labor.

Roni asks if I am complaining that she does not spend enough time taking care of the babies. "No," I say, but the look on her face says we both know I am lying. Roni's feelings are hurt. "You know how hard it is for me to wake up," Roni says. She has always suffered from insomnia, but once she's asleep, she is gone. I could roll sushi on her back when she is sleeping. Roni can barely crawl out of bed in the morning.

"I wish I could be the one waking up with the babies," Roni says. "I wish I could see them smiling and googling in the morning instead of fighting for a seat on the train."

Sometimes, when I walk a crying baby in the middle of

the night in the hallway, I see Roni roll over and crack one eye open. I scurry down to the end of the hall, worried I have interrupted her sleep, but now it dawns on me that what I am really afraid of is seeing the silent regret in Roni's eyes that she is not in the hallway, taking care of her babies, their infancy disappearing under oceans of paperwork.

Neither one of us planned for this arrangement. Roni and I never expected to become involved, get married, or have kids together. We only started dating to break out of our monotonous dating habits. That was the only thing we had in common. We didn't even like each other.

Roni and I met in 1990, when I was a senior editor at Film Tech, making $40,000 a year and living in an illegal sublet. I ducked the landlord by pretending I was the lover of Katherine M., the fifty-something woman I sublet from, a former Ziegfeld girl who was divorced from a Spanish bullfighter and traveled around the world like the last Bohemian. Katherine kept all her life's possessions in towering, seven-foot-high stacks of blue Bloomingdale's gift boxes, which took up half the floor space of the apartment and drove everyone who visited me berserk with curiosity, but which I never opened, not once in seven years. The stucco walls were painted dark blue, and the place was as dark as an insane asylum.

I worked, ate dinner with friends in cheap restaurants, and dated an assortment of women who were, in retrospect, clinically insane. I specialized in aspiring actresses, each of whom was more self-absorbed and self-hating than the last. I jogged up and down the stairs in the five-floor walk-up building because I couldn't afford a health club. The elderly residents reacted with fright as I grunted past them.

At work, I read the sex column in a free newspaper while eating my lunch—other people's sex problems always struck me as hilarious—which appeared inside the personal ads. One week the paper ran a special in which anyone could place a personal ad for free, with free voice messages, so, on a whim, I submitted an ad.

"Men are jerks," I wrote. "Selfish, self-absorbed, insensitive, bad listeners, inflexible. SWM, none of the above, seeks SWF who defies all clichés."

Of the twenty-five or so responses, Roni's was shuffled to the bottom of the list because she was a lawyer. Also, Roni left a message "for Ed number three hundred and seventy-one"—she was really saying "Ad number three hundred and seventy-one," but I misheard it—and worried she was psychotic. Who was Ed? And what happened to the first 370 of him? I finally called her after burning through about twenty-two or twenty-three vaguely nightmarish dates. By the end I had streamlined it down to assembly-line, ten-minute coffee dates. I was growing more focused on creating a well-oiled dating system than actually meeting a woman.

Roni and her girlfriend Nancy circled personal ads in newspapers and magazines and critiqued them as a hobby, but never answered any. My satirical, Rohrschach-y ad made Roni laugh, so Nancy badgered her to call me.

Roni wore a T-shirt, jeans with a foot-high cuff, and work boots to the first date. I wore black jeans and a black T-shirt, turned inside out for reasons that seemed appropriate at the time. We had no chemistry at all, and the conversation was extremely stilted. I remember Roni telling a story about capturing cockroaches and setting them on fire (a story she now denies). We were bored and unimpressed with each other, but, ironically, each of us had vowed privately to date outside our usual-suspects list. So I called her a week later and we had a boring movie date. She called me one week later, and we had a boring bike-riding date. We stuck with it and dated once a week, as if taking an antibiotic regimen. Our weirdnesses seem to fit. We had sympathetic dysfunctions.

What attracted me to Roni was that, in New York, a city of pretenders and poseurs, she was that rare thing: a hard-core eccentric. She loved hardware stores and wildflowers and vintage clothes, and was never so happy as when she bought something cool at a tag sale for two dollars, even if she didn't need it, or it was too big to move, or an environmental hazard. Roni reminded me of women I had met in small towns in Virginia or Vermont or Texas, women who said what they felt and didn't care what men, or even other women, thought of them. Neither Roni nor I really fit in to New York City life. Roni was real—weird, but real, and that was sexy.

Roni says she fell for me because I was a good listener, I wasn't critical, I didn't try to change her or box her in, and I was thoughtful. The first time she blurted out "I love you" was when I called from my local Laundromat to say I was bringing chicken soup across town to help knock back her cold.

We never discussed our income disparity. She owned an apartment and I moved in, even though it was half-gutted and looked like an abandoned construction site.

We didn't discuss money until we planned the wedding,

which we paid for, since her parents, both retired, had no savings, my dad had been in debt from his stock market gambling since I was a small child, and my mom, now in her sixties, worked at GMAC, processing mortgages for maybe $17,000 a year and struggling to pay her bills.

When we learned we couldn't have children, and that we needed to enroll in an in-vitro fertilization program, which cost about $10,000 per cycle, we both sold off our 401(K)s and borrowed the rest.

We didn't discuss money again until Asher was born and we had to decide if I would quit my job and stay home or go to work and hire a nanny, who would eat up 90 percent of my take-home salary. We decided I should keep working and look for a better job.

And so we dedicated ourselves to protecting Roni's job, which means that I took over the grunt work. When Asher had stomach viruses and his explosive diarrhea spread over the bed and the changing table and the floor, I stayed up for hours sanitizing the apartment and snuggling him back down to sleep. One day I picked him up from a play date where he ate pizza and grape juice, and in the taxi he got sick. We were going 30 and the driver couldn't hear me yelling to stop, so I caught Asher's voluminous jet-stream vomit in my bare hands and shirt and heaved it out the taxi's window onto Amsterdam Avenue. I woke in the dead of the night for every little problem, and early every morning. I sang dumb songs when I diapered him and we invented dopey games to get dressed and clean up and stay busy on rainy days. Asher and I are connected because I was always there to take care of him. Children demand immediate attention, in the middle of the night, in the middle of a meal, in the middle of a phone call, always impossibly inconveniently in the middle of something else, and I am more naturally suited to this pressure. Sometimes Roni joked that I was Asher's slave, but for the first few years, slavery is an accurate job description.

Roni missed most of Asher's early childhood, working until 1:00 or 2:00 in the morning every night and sleeping helplessly until noon on weekends. She doesn't mention this unless we are deep in the middle of a fight, and then she unleashes it, disguised as an angry offensive attack. But when the dust settles I know she said it defensively, out of pain and loss. It is a raw emotion I avoid out of guilt, because being dad to Asher means more to me than any job, and my most frustrating day at home with Asher was fifty times better than my best day at work, and in the shifting math of the household equations, the numbers are on my side.

So I take pride in my exhaustion, knowing it is a gift I will not fully appreciate until later. I am a night warrior. I can wake from a dead sleep and pluck a crying baby from his or her crib in less than ten seconds' elapsed time. I can sense a wet bed with the psychic accuracy Stephen King could build a novel around. I know which cough means nothing and which cough will produce a crying, feverish child, looking for love.

The night is no longer some magical, mystical territory that defines the border between days. The night is just another day, a dark day, slipped in between. I am with my kids at night, watching over them, anticipating their needs.

About six months later, when I go to Los Angeles on a business trip, I will sleep with the lights, TV, and radio on, unable to adjust to the eerie, suffocating silence of the three-star hotel room. I will wake up every hour, my heart racing with the panic that something has gone terribly wrong. A crying child is as natural to me as my own breathing. The absence of crying is abnormal, and I could not sleep for eight straight hours if I wanted. The old oceanlike realms of deep sleep are so unnatural that I would feel as if I were drowning, and wake up, shaking in terror.

SEVEN

The Worry-Go-Round

Bronxville reminds me of Riverdale, the town from the Archie comics I read religiously as a nine-year-old. The village, population 6,500, exists in a Betty and Veronica time warp where blue-eyed, blond-haired boys and girls walk to the old schoolhouse bearing dry-cleaned backpacks, silver-haired old ladies strategically occupy public benches and broker the daily gossip, and the bakery wraps up its pastries in white boxes and string. The moms are tall and thin and blond and sport teeth like baby grand piano keys. The husbands look like they were born on the eighteenth green of a Master's PGA tour.

The babies are seven weeks old now. We have been in the new house just a week. We live near the railroad station, where a few dilapidated A-frame houses are available for rent. No new housing has been built in Bronxville Village since World War II and the stately, *Metropolitan Home*-ready, Tudor Colonials carry a median price tag of about $1 million. We were lucky to find an affordable four-bedroom house to rent here, even if it is falling apart. But it is a good house for us, with a dining room, living room, even a tiny front and backyard. The idea is to live here for two years while we write a new master plan.

The day we moved in, Roni frowned with buyer's remorse. "It's smaller than I thought," she said. She stared vacantly around the living room, as if she had shown up at the wrong wedding.

Imprisoned in bed rest, Roni never saw her new home with her own eyes before moving in, but only through my amateur videotapes. The rooms looked smaller because of the way video distorts space. The paint was fifteen years old and peeling, the kitchen linoleum was from the 1930s, and I conveniently left out the part about Audrey, the sweet, sixty-something retired librarian who lived on the third floor above us in a converted granny flat with half a dozen cats. We heard Audrey clomping up and down the stairs and the cats spinning and scrambling furiously around her.

"It will be nice to have someone around in case of emergencies," I tried.

"I smell cat," Roni said.

"Don't complain," said Ima, who drove down from Schenectady with Abba. I couldn't decide if my mother-in-law was more critical of me behind my back or to my wife right to her face.

"A house is a house," Ima said.

Abba wandered around the house muttering about what a piece of crap it was. They were tough, intelligent, resilient people, my in-laws, and they considered me a kind of harmless moron because I was a writer and their daughter had been duped into providing the bulk of the family income. Of course, Roni picked me of her own free will, so she was knocked down a couple of pegs herself.

"We're only renting it," I said. "We couldn't afford to stay in the city."

We adjust to the house. Late at night I end up down in the basement, which is dark and dingy but to me miraculous: A whole, separate universe for nonessentials, extras, junk, spillovers, unsortables. Finally, separation between our stuff and us.

Instead of living with boxes stacked all around us, like angry ghosts, the boxes will live in the basement, among themselves. When I find some object that does not meet an immediate need it is dispatched right down into the basement instead of bouncing around for weeks. We don't have to live imprisoned by objects. All these boxes labeled Misc.—an envelope of old birthday cards, orphaned pieces of toys, a duplicate garlic press, a bag of antique hardware for a French door we don't have anymore but which is too valuable to toss out, the half-finished roll of wrapping paper, a stack of expired coupons, a manual to an answering machine—right down to the basement, without a trial, without due process, without a hearing. When I packed up the apartment, Roni yelled from bed, "I want to know what's going in all those boxes!" I took an almost erotic pleasure in unceremoniously consigning Roni's crazy junk into boxes. I scribbled notes about anything that might prove useful in the future—a bag of nice antique buttons, a left-handed pair of scissors, a copy of her law school application.

Now, standing amid all our boxes, I have vivid memories of my childhood basement and all my great stuff—my books and baseball cards and train sets and my souped-up electric slot cars, rewired by my crazy uncle Harold, my dad's best friend, who died of stomach cancer when I was sixteen. My boxes of comic books—Archie, Sad Sack, Little Lotta, Richie Rich, Ripley's Believe It or Not. Where did they all go? Did we give it all away or throw it in the garbage? Is some kid in Pennsylvania playing with my old train set? How did Roni and I survive for five years in the city without a basement?

"What are you doing down in the basement?" Roni yells down.

"Nothing," I say, a bit guiltily. Just thinking.

I race home from the city by 7:00 or 7:30 to relieve Rosetta and her friend Agnes, who now works for us part-time. I am on my own with Asher and the triplets until Roni returns home between 10:00 and 12:00, unless she is working on a deal, which means 1:00, 2:00, even 3:00 A.M. Sometimes, when I leave the babies' room in the middle of the night, Roni and I collide on the second floor landing, shocked to find the other person in our midst.

Roni is obsessed with subduing the spreading chaos of our lives. She redesigns the closet in the babies' nursery, builds special shelves, buys plastic containers to store the sheets, onesies, clothes, sleepy hats. She folds and refolds the baby clothes until the edges are razor sharp. The pantry is packed and repacked for greatest ergonomic ease. Roni scours tag sales to find household odds and ends for which she refuses to pay retail. Shopping trips are diagrammed like military assaults.

All this orchestrating and coordinating leaves me alone with the kids on the weekends. In between playing, shopping, cooking, and cleaning, I change twenty-five to thirty diapers a day. On three-day holiday weekends, Tuesday morning looms across an ocean of bottles and burps and diaper pails like a distant star. "You're better at it than I am," Roni says. "You *like* changing diapers."

A larger design is working itself out. Roni makes the strategic decisions and I execute. She picks Asher's school, I fill out the forms. She decides the menu for Thanksgiving, I shop for the ingredients, clean the kitchen, move around the furniture. She buys living room furniture and changes her mind, I return it and argue with the store manager.

Roni is right about the diapers, although I wouldn't say I enjoy changing diapers as much as find it oddly satisfying. Writing a screenplay takes years, and is never really over, but a clean diaper is a personal, handmade victory that can be achieved five or ten times a day. What can be more satisfying than knowing your kid is clean and dry and happy and you're the only one in the world capable?

Roni is transferring some of her unhappiness with our economic situation into folding and planning and bossing me around. I can live with that. But I am distressed over Roni's increasingly narrow and obsessive behavior.

Roni has always shown obsessive-compulsive tendencies. She sometimes counts floors in building we are entering. If a room isn't left a certain way she can't leave the house. But she is a split-personality control freak. She will organize the baby's nursery down to the last inch, but our bedroom is left fallow, to turn into an epic disaster of clutter, baby toys and shopping bags and dirty clothes everywhere. I find weeks-old, half-eaten sandwiches on the bed, power tools, office files, crumpled Visa card receipts. From time to time the cordless phone will be lost for days, turning up inside a cloverleaf of bedcovers and dirty laundry and wilted newspaper sections.

"I'm getting to the bedroom," Roni says. In Roni's mind, a project designated for completion occupies the same mental space as a project actually completed. Roni does not see the bedroom as dirty and in disarray. Instead, she sees the bedroom of the future, as it should be. But I am sleeping on a bag of stockings and socks and hair bows that need to be returned to a store that has gone out of business.

"Kind of like when you talk about your career as a comedy writer, but I'm still working ninety hours a week?" Roni says.

"I have to go down to the basement," I say.

Roni and I are not smart fighters. We tend to go nuclear when attacked, rather than analyze what is really upsetting the other person. We are both under tremendous pressure. Aside from the bed rest, Roni has no wiggle room at work. When a deal is being done, she stays up all night to make sure the printer executes the offering properly and the SEC receives the required documents. The senior corporate partners may suddenly jump all over the smallest details of a deal. Roni receives no domestic slack whatsoever and cannot even ask for time off to go to the pediatrician. If the trains run slow and she arrives at 9:01 for the 9:00 corporate meeting, she is berated.

I am juggling so many different masters—Asher, the babies, the nannies, Nicky, Roni, and the house—that I feel lost. Sometimes I find myself on the porch with my car keys in my hand and no idea whether I am leaving or arriving, if groceries need to go into the refrigerator or a child is waiting to be picked up.

When one of us explodes it is like a blast in a weapons dump—the other one always explodes, too. Sometimes Roni says she wants to get divorced, and my reaction is to say fine, as long as I get the kids, and then she says I only care about the children and that's the whole problem, and then we fight about the future terms of our theoretical divorce, down to who will pay for the furniture in the second house and who is emotionally mature enough to determine what day is treat day.

Roni is not the introspective type—she is as much a mystery to herself as she is to me—and I study her like a piece of abstract art to figure out why she is angry. Sometimes this backfires, though, like the night she is angry about a pot left in the sink with no water in it.

"There must be something else bothering you. You can't be that angry about the stupid pot," I say.

No, just the fact that she has told me a thousand times to fill the pots with water so the dirt doesn't cake on. Even though I am the one doomed to wash the pot later that night, the wanton disregard for the condition of the pot—not to mention her express wish that the pots not be abandoned—drives her crazy.

Her anger over the pot drives me insane with its surface pettiness, but if I take several large steps back, I can see the invisible thread that runs through such fights. The water in the pot, the garbage bag left on the porch, the drips of oatmeal that hardened on the dining room table—these cracks in the system are symbols of chaos descending and swallowing us, especially when she walks in the front door at 11:45 P.M., exhausted and demoralized, to find the latest domestic anomalies. When she attacks me for the pot in the sink I am furious because she ignores the one hundred other chores I completed that day. She overlooks some of my grunt work, but she is trapped in her office when she would rather be home, and even if she kept the house like a war zone at least it would be her war zone. I tell her we need a maid twice a week, but she can't stand a stranger cleaning the house, because that is tantamount to a complete surrender of her house-mistressing status. So I tell myself not to argue when she complains that the newspaper in the recycling bin is stacked improperly. It's not the newspaper. It's not the newspaper, I tell myself.

"What's not the newspaper?!" Roni says, looking at me suspiciously, as she bends angrily over the recycling box.

Was that an audible? "Nothing," I say.

At the same time, Roni and I are deeply connected. One night Roni is working in the bedroom at about 11:30, but dozing off. Asher is asleep and I am feeding the babies. I lay Jared in the bassinet and run downstairs to fill a bottle for him, because he is crying and fussing. I fumble around in the kitchen, cursing as drying bottles and nipples scatter to the floor, when I hear something peculiar—silence. I listen for a second, and race back up the stairs to find Roni standing in the hallway with a strange look on her face.

She points into the nursery, where I see Asher, sitting on the floor, gently pulling Jared into his lap and comforting him.

"Shhh, Jawie, it's okay," Asher says. "Daddy's bringing your baba. Shh—don't cry. Daddy makes a good baba, right?"

I see Jared's round little face turned up toward Asher, transfixed. Roni and I look at each other and smile like teenage lovers. I put my arm around her. We don't say a word, just watch Asher and Jared for a few minutes, until I realize the bottle is overheating on the stove, and may possibly explode, and race back downstairs. Roni yells down and asks me to bring her a cookie on the return trip. "Me, too!" Asher pipes up. Cookies for everyone!

Roni has a major folding disorder. I tease her about it, even in front of friends and family, because she appears to be at peace over it, and it's not as if she needs to attend weekly meetings or take medication. In fact, given all my anxieties, I should be thankful Roni's one neuroses is about housekeeping.

One night I wake at 2:00 A.M. to the sound of Roni sighing apocalyptically. She is burning through the hallway linen closet, methodically refolding every single towel. When I do the laundry I put the towels away the quick and manly way—fold them in half, then half again. Roni cannot bear to look at this squared-off version of a towel, stacked with floppy, sloppy folds facing unforgivably in four different directions. Roni folds the towel lengthwise into thirds, then over itself in half, creating one large, soft, con-tiguous rounded side that faces outward when stacked. The towels look like props in a fabric-softener TV commercial. Sometimes I find Roni refolding all the kid's clothing in one of the drawers, mumbling to herself.

"I think you fold the towels the wrong way just to drive me crazy," Roni says. I tell her that if I wanted to gaslight her, I would be more creative—and faster.

Roni needs to take the folding thing down a notch. She is unhappy at work—her boss is ten times the control freak she is, and nothing drives a control freak crazier than to be subject to the alien mindscape of another control freak—and she feels she will never assume dominion over the house.

The relentless folding and refolding, the endless shopping trips, the restacking of the pantry, are desperate attempts to seize back a feeling of power. But our life is out of control for a while, and we will have to lean into the wave and body surf to wherever it is we are going. You can't control the future. You can't control the past. You can barely control the next five minutes.

"That's a stupid analogy, and you know how much I hate water," Roni says.

"Just do what she says, no matter how crazy it sounds," says my friend and marital-issue consigliere Michael Billig. "Smile and do it her way. Save your energy for the big battles."

"I always liked Michael," Roni says.

My mom calls to say she is worried about me, about the stress, given that I am not volunteering enough information. I can't tell her I am worried, too, because I worry how she will worry. She is also worried about Asher: Is he being forgotten? Do I have enough time to spend with him? Is he jealous of the babies? Is Roni being hard on him?

I reassure her that Asher is doing well in school and that our home life is like a birthday party. I don't want my mother to worry, because this is my job description now, and it would be a redundant use of personnel. I instruct my mom to consider herself retired from the worrying racket. Her new job is life chancellor. But it cracks me up when I fuss over the same crazy details with the kids that my mother still worries about me. We ride the same parental worry-go-round.

EIGHT

My Fifteen Minutes

To make one grandiose mark on our new life, Roni bought a massive Italian stroller—used, because she hated to pay full price—from another mother of triplets. It took me six hours to disassemble the contraption in the basement of the woman's apartment building, haul it to the street in pieces, stuff it in the Suburban, and drive it to the new house. I lost two weeks—and two pints of blood—in the reassembly.

The babies are eight weeks old now. We have been in the new house two weeks. The new stroller looks like the bastard child of a Victorian baby pram and the Brooklyn Bridge, with intersecting crossbars topped by four massive sea blue seats with retractable hoods. The vehicle is a colorful and impractical monstrosity, completely lacking in basic engineering. None of the wheels turn—they are on a wheelbarrow-style axle—which makes it like pushing a piano. I lift up the back wheels whenever I need to turn.

Loaded with babies, the stroller weighs one hundred and fifty awkwardly distributed pounds.

The sidewalk running from our house into town is a steep downgrade that passes a two-hundred-year-old Catholic church. When I stop in front of the church to make an adjustment, I invite the very real possibility of running myself over.

"Like in the Road Runner cartoon, the way Coyote always dies," I explain to Roni. We are out on the sidewalk, testing the stroller.

"Isn't it amazing?" Roni says, her face lit up like a full moon.

"I hate it. It's ridiculous," I say. "We'll never use it. We'll hang towels on it."

"Daddy, stop saying mean things about Mommy's carriage!" Asher scolds, his round, angelic face squaring off into an angry exclamation point. This is highly momentous, Asher taking his mother's side. As the house disciplinarian, she rarely enjoys his sanctuary.

"I'll put the snow suits on the babies!" Roni says. "You two boys take them for a test spin. Sound like fun?" She gives Asher a conspiratorial squeeze.

"Sure!" Asher says, smiling after his mother. He turns to me with disapproving eyes.

"Oh, great," I say, as Roni dashes into the house with her awkward girlie steps. When she is dorky and excited and full of goofy enthusiasm, I act like Ralph Cramden on the outside, but my heart quietly leaps.

"Stop it!" Asher says.

The first few weeks in the new house, Roni is too exhausted to do anything besides boil water and endlessly rearrange baby clothes, so Asher and I make the early journeys together. One day he holds the carriage while I tighten a front wheel, weighing the force of his attention span against the laws of gravity.

Asher understands the runaway stroller's destructive trajectory, the lights snapping on in his busy little head. He tests his grip on the carriage, holding the handlebar with four fingers, then three, then two.

"Uh-oh," he says, pretending to let go.

He asks if we can set the carriage free, to see what will happen. I scold him for this idea as I smile secretly over its evil precocity. How much damage would the sea blue behemoth actually inflict (without babies, of course) running headlong into, say, that blue Ford Explorer? Do I think like my three-year-old, or does my three-year-old think like an adult?

After a week, I grudgingly admit to Roni that I can pile the babies into the stroller in one-third the time it takes to strap them into the car. Three minutes later, I will be slugging down my Starbucks coffee, one of the fringe benefits of living in a self-contained village.

"Say you were wrong," Roni says, putting her face in front of mine. Roni is romantically aroused when I admit I am wrong.

"You were wrong," I say.

"Daddy!" Asher says.

The first time Asher and I take the babies out around Bronxville is a warm day in late March and the babies are eight weeks old. We roll down past the church, cross the street with the supermarket and Chinese take-out restaurant, and parade the babies through the **V**-shaped heart of the village.

The reaction is instantaneous. The Bronxville locals literally stop in their tracks and stare at us. Heads turn. Cars slow down. Drivers honk their horns and wave. People stop and formally introduce themselves.

The strategy behind this ridiculous stroller looks prophetic. Roni's desire to show the babies off to the world was so simple, and so obvious, that I missed it completely. People flock around Asher and me, peppering us with personal questions. Are they twins? They can't possibly be triplets? Were you on fertility drugs? Why don't they look alike? What are the names?

To become an overnight celebrity is disorienting. After just a few days, hundreds of people know my name and remember conversations, personal facts or tidbits of my history. On every corner I hear the constant soft whispering, "There goes the father. . . ."

The attention of our new neighbors is unbelievably earnest. No sarcasm, no sniping, no cynical put-downs, just heartfelt compliments. Bronxville is three miles from the New York City border but a hundred years behind in the cynicism department. Stay-at-home moms in Bronxville don't do irony. They do ironing.

I am proud of my family and the shot of celebrity feels good. Over the last twenty years I did stand-up comedy, sold jokes to comedians, wrote scripts for TV shows and movies, wrote short stories, stage plays, screenplays, and novels, with little success. My fifteen minutes of fame are finally here.

. . .

One morning I shove the baby tank into Starbucks, blasting paint off the door frame. "Hi, Dad!" waves Claire, one of the high school barista girls. The Starbucks people know me, generically, as Dad. I am a reliable source of amusement with my bouncing plastic bottles, Ziploc bag of baby formula, bag of ointments and Band-aids and burpie towels.

Today I catch the attention of an overly tanned forty-something woman, inappropriately dressed as a teenager—high heels, leopardskin stretch pants, four-inch red nails. I recognize her as a regular. She gabs with the girls behind the counter.

"Are they all yours?" the overtanned woman asks.

The babies are fraternal, not identical, so the question is vaguely within the realm of logic, although it indicates a personality more prone to leaping than looking.

"Yes," I say. "They're triplets."

"Well," the overtanned woman says, her face collecting into a surgically altered frown. "I'm glad it's not me," she whispers, winking at one of the Starbucks girls.

"Boy, I'm glad, too!" I say, very, very, very loudly, smiling like a hyena.

The overtanned woman stops, her arm on the door, lipstick-smeared coffee cup frozen in midair. She senses this is an insult.

I feel like a million dollars as the dragon lady leaves in a froth of confusion. How many times in my life have I delivered the perfect insult during the actual incident? How many times have I tossed and turned at night, wishing

I could have said what I wanted to say after hours of mental editing?

"God bless you!" says a muscular, tattooed, very handsome Cuban man, about twenty-seven. It is a few days after the Starbucks incident. The man is walking to a construction site and stops dead in his steel-toe-booted tracks when he sees the three babies and Asher.

"You're a real man!" he gushes, pointing to the carriage. "Taking care of three little babies. That's for *real*." He says something in Spanish, another compliment, which I do not understand. He gently shakes Asher's hand. Asher smiles nervously and holds on to my leg. He is a city kid, unfamiliar with this level of enthusiasm.

The young man crushes my hand in his terrifying Golden Gloves grip, says a blessing over the babies in Spanish, then rushes off to his work site, turning to wave at us with his bulging lats and deltoids.

I am speechless. I thought I had developed a thick skin about these public encounters, but I am still continually surprised by the emotional weight of people's reactions. The attention offsets the casual hostility I endure at work. Nicky is a divorced, childless, mid-forties guy with a large bushy mustache and a taste for cowboy boots and black jeans. He is a boisterous backslapper and hand shaker and drink buyer. He is a chart flipper and a reader of motivational books and loves sales conventions and sales guys who beat their quotas. To his credit, our magazine is his family, and he is the pathologically loyal company man. In his world, babies, due to their inability to place 12X ad contracts or buy four-color inserts, are simply useless.

Only one other person in my office has kids, but they are grown. So I am a corporate anomaly. When I rush back from lunch, dragging bags of diapers and wipes, my co-workers roll their eyes. We have a nanny, so there is confusion over why I must run errands or visit the pediatrician. In the corporate environment, other people's babies are an annoyance at best and a danger to the bottom line at worst.

But in Bronxville, complete strangers grab me by the shoulders to tell me "God bless you!" Women kiss me on both cheeks. Men grab my hand and congratulate me as if I just ran a game-winning touchdown. Women clutch their hands to their chests and tell me how lucky I am, how blessed my family is. I always reply that we *are* blessed. Even after I say it one hundred times, it does not feel routine.

One Sunday morning I walk past the Catholic church as early mass lets out. The priest is on the steps in his green vestments, saying good-bye to his flock, and the sidewalk is crowded and noisy, five deep.

"Excuse me, coming through," I say, ice breaking through the milling flock. The priest sees the commotion and, after learning about the triplets, recites a blessing over them. The crowd bubbles with excitement. Old ladies pinch Asher on the cheek. "The big brother!" they say. Old men in hound's-tooth jackets and dentures slap me on the arm.

Roni has not basked in this local glory. Exhausted and shaken from the C-section, the debilitating bed rest, and the return to her brutal work schedule, she sleeps late Saturday and Sunday mornings. Finally, in early April, Roni

travels with us one Saturday morning. We reach the Starbucks, turn right, and the first crowd gathers.

"God bless you!" says a woman, who stops and chats for
fifteen minutes. Finally, I break it up with a carefully
timed, "We have to get these babies rolling."

Roni glares at me. "You don't understand," I explain.
"You have your public to think of." We don't move more
than a few feet when we are stopped by a group of five
older men and women.

"God bless your family," says one of the men. They fire
questions at us, adding commentary about who the babies
look like, feeding advice, even decorating tips. "Buy
couches and rugs with dark, mixed patterns that hide
stains," one of the women says.

"Eleanor was a decorator," explains the woman's husband. "She's allergic to wheat."

Roni is elated by the God-bless-yous. "That's a million
blessings!" she says.

I pretend to be skeptical. "They say the same thing if
you sneeze," I say.

I described the town's reaction to the babies, but to feel
it in person is overwhelming. Roni's eyes shimmer with
excitement as she gossips and shows off and connects with
the other moms, some of whom met me before and won-
dered what Roni would be like. Roni's smile is so wide I
see teeth I never knew existed. She is floating on air. I
could put a string on her leg and fly her around like a kite.

"This is the big brother!" Roni says to an elderly woman.
The pride in Roni's voice is so crisp and clear that Asher
shrinks back in embarrassment.

Underneath her excitement is a well of sadness. Roni
wants to push the kids around town and show off her tribe,

and the injustice hurts. She nurtured them and carried them to term and gambled her life for them, and now her reward is to be locked up in her office ninety hours a week and sleep half the weekend away just to feel normal on Monday morning. I reschedule the weekends to do the grocery shopping in the morning and the walking tours in the afternoon, when Roni has more energy. Bronxville is only a few blocks square, but Roni plans our weekend jaunts on Friday night as though we were tackling a week in Paris or London.

It is hard not to feel optimistic about humanity when strangers line up two deep to bless you and proclaim how extraordinary you and your children are. But enough bizarre and intrusive questions are sprinkled in to keep the process unpredictable.

"You must be exhausted," a fortyish woman says as we swing past the toy store.

"Yes," I say. "They don't sleep very much."

"It must be hard for you and your wife to have . . . private time," the woman says.

I am not sure what she is talking about, exactly, but her body language suggests the acute possibility of a sexual subtext. Something about this woman looks a little bit off center, so I check Asher for his reaction. He is highly intuitive and is my canary in the mineshaft of human complexity. Asher regards this woman with tight lips and hooded eyes, so I hurry us away.

"They must eat quite a lot," says a white-haired businessman near the train station one evening. He wears an expensive English suit, immaculate wing tips, and French cuffs. His buttery leather briefcase costs more than my salary for two months.

He is running a spreadsheet in his head—four kids, at three meals a day, seven days a week—

"We're lucky," I say. "They are extremely good eaters."

This throws him. He smiles politely but forgoes follow-up questions. This category of inquiry—the tonnage of baby food required, the cost of maintenance—grows rapidly in the mental pie chart I maintain of frequently asked questions.

"How do you know they're triplets?" asks an elderly woman one night. She seems confused. I briefly outline the in-vitro fertilization process, but this only increases the woman's anxiety, and she retreats before I reach the word "blastocyst."

Many of the comments relate to our luck at winning the fertility lottery. Often, people trying to sound empathetic impart a strange negative subtext.

"That's a lot of kids," a woman says one night. "I mean—really a lot."

"That must be really difficult," another woman says.

"I feel for you," a man says.

"Cheaper by the dozen!" I say. "One pregnancy is better than three!"

A friendly woman puts her hand on my shoulder one day. Her son is whining and kicking at her foot. "I don't know how you do it," she says. "I only have two kids, and I'm ready to shoot myself."

.   .   .

It is spring now, a warm Sunday in late April. The babies are three months old. I sit on a bench with Asher, eating bagels. The babies take little dog naps next to us.

Asher is working on a muffin, a secret muffin, of which his carbohydrate-busting mother would disapprove. My pleasure in Asher's enjoyment of the unlawful muffin goes a long way in explaining my emotional immaturity and our combative marriage.

An older couple walks past us, stops at the butcher shop, and turns to stare. The husband walks with a limp and wears a floppy ribbed fishing hat. I am used to the staring and explain that they are triplets.

"Why don't they all look the same?" the woman asks. She seems dissatisfied, almost suspicious, of my boilerplate explanation.

"All twins are identical," she tells her husband. "Even if they don't look the same." The woman eyes the babies, trying to comprehend the fraud I am perpetrating.

"They're all *different*," chimes in Asher. He puts his muffin down and looks at me, indignant. The woman's hostility infuriates him. Asher has become increasingly protective of the babies in public. When kids try to touch the babies, Asher puts his body in between them and the carriage, body-blocking them. I don't know where he learned this technique. He hasn't turned three yet.

"See," Asher says, pointing to Barak. "This one has blond hair. Barak. *B* for *blond* hair! See?" I let Asher continue, and the woman eventually retreats, unburdened by any clearer picture of the phenomenon she has just seen.

Asher sits down, takes a bite of his muffin, and sighs expressively, like a public school teacher who has delivered another lesson to a class that is not paying attention.

"Some people," I say.

"Have you started thinking about college?" asks a woman with a tall, gangly teenage daughter in tow. I am outside the Food Emporium, battening down the hatches for a supermarket adventure.

"We're just trying to get some sleep," I say.

"Seriously," the woman says. "My sister has three kids, and her husband is a CPA, and he says they need to put away one hundred and fifty thousand dollars in cash now, at nine percent, to pay for college, and not Ivy League college." She accents every other word for emphasis.

"Wow," I say. "Hmmm!" I manufacture a story about a Lucky Charms coupon expiring and hurry into the supermarket. If my wife and I can live in total denial of the financial tsunami bearing down upon us, who is this woman to splash cold water in my face?

I ease into my role as celebrity dad. I have heard all the questions now. I know which jokes work on what demographic segment and how to cut a conversation short politely. I can handle three confused old ladies like Bob Barker.

One night we are outside Starbucks so Asher can walk the "balance beam," the two-inch rock ledge that encloses the landscaping. It is a busy intersection across from the train station, and I see people whose names, faces, jobs, and family situations are familiar.

A tall, gazellelike woman with wide-spaced eyes, towering a foot above me, obviously a runway model, stops dead in her tracks.

"Wow!" she says. Her eyes move from one baby to the next. She is young, maybe twenty or twenty-one, stunningly beautiful and unselfconscious, except for the tightly wound, 35-ish boyfriend, who sports five-day stubble and designer sunglasses parked over gelled-back hair. The boyfriend grips her elbow tensely and hustles her inside with a sour look in my direction. The last thing this guy needs is a chitchat about babies.

Later that day, a nattily dressed, silver-haired man, right off the cover of *Forbes,* along with his equally turned-out wife, breeze by us. The wife says, "That reminds me, we have to call Sylvana about the Three Tenors show."

One demand of even minor celebrityhood is a memory for names, faces, and biographical details. In this respect I am also a failure. One day at the Bronxville train station, a strange woman touches my arm.

"You were right about the neighbors," the strange woman says. I smile back, dumbfounded. Have I been bad-mouthing my neighbors, the sweet couple from Brazil? Is there another neighbor I have spoken out against? I am mortified that I might have acted like some snobby New York loudmouth.

The woman and I chat about the weather. I can't begin to guess about her job, kids, husband, house. The train arrives and we board together. I am terrified she will sit next to me, so I excuse myself and look for the bathroom, even though we both know the train has no bathrooms.

In the Bronxville video store a few weeks later it hits me. I was in here with the kids and chatted with this woman about how much I loved the John Belushi and Dan Akroyd comedy, *Neighbors*. The woman didn't say I was right about "the neighbors," but *Neighbors*.

Some days I wonder if I have been wrong to measure Bronxville against our experience in Manhattan. What would our life be like if we lived in one of the small towns I spent time in, like Traverse City, Michigan, or Waxahachie, Texas? Would we be cherished local celebrities, with people baking cakes and offering to baby-sit—two gestures no one here has dared to make—or would we be town weirdos? I lean to the thought that we would have a refrigerator full of smoked brisket and BBQ chicken, a trunkful of homemade quilts, and teenage baby-sitters packed into the living room if we lived in Texas.

If the population of Bronxville is 6,500, I calculate that, after a few months, most of the full-time residents will greet me at least once. Therefore, the novelty of my appearance should begin to level off as we reach the far side of the bell curve.

As usual with things mathematical, I am wrong. By early May, when the babies are thirteen weeks old, no change in the rate of comments can be observed. But the comments begin to fall into predictable patterns, as people form psychographic clusters.

"They don't look like you," says a young woman with a dog.

"Congratulations. They look just like you," says a young mother, pushing a stroller, minutes later. These two women belong to the Genetics Cluster. Some of the comments in the Genetics Cluster prove puzzling. If the babies "look like me," is that always a compliment? If so, is it a compliment to me or the babies? And if resembling me is a compliment, is it an automatic insult if the babies do not look like me?

With a gradual decline in God-bless-yous, the Genetics Cluster overtakes the Religious Cluster. As the babies grow, sprout hair, sit up, and look different, the old, pure "God Bless You" slips down the greatest-hits chart. Apparently, three slightly broken-in babies are less deserving of divine protection than three newborns.

"I guess you can get used to anything," says a woman with patches sewn onto her blue-jeans dress. She is in the Unconscious Hostility Cluster.

"If they're healthy, that's what counts," says a thin woman, 50-ish, with a voice like Nick Nolte. She falls within the Philosophy Lite Cluster.

"Wow, I thought I had it tough," says a mom pushing twins. We exchange diaper, bottle, sleeping, and eating trivia. This is the Foxhole Bonding Cluster, my favorite. I am a giant Acme-cartoon magnet for moms with twins. If I sold life insurance, real estate, or time shares, I could retire on my moms-with-twins accounts.

One day a haggard-looking woman stops near us to rummage through her bag. She is pushing a stroller with a crying baby boy, fifteen or sixteen months old. He is restless, colicky.

I am teasing my babies, stealing their milk bottles and pretending to drink them. Asher is playing along and we are laughing, making a spectacle.

"Hah!" the woman says, looking at me. I cannot tell if

she is thinking out loud, trying to provoke a response, or suffering a breakdown in her meds, but her eyes are black from lack of sleep and she has a sad, defeated look that makes me feel sorry.

"It's a lot of work, isn't it?" I say. The woman looks me up and down, at the way Asher interacts with the babies, and her shoulders soften. The black cloud hovering above her head breaks up a bit.

"Yeah," she says. "Well, good luck," she adds, and crosses the street, heading for the video store. I hear her baby's angry squalling for another two blocks. Where is the Superdad Groupie Cluster, anyway?

The truly insane and demented questions are entertaining as sociological feedback. "Do they have any pets?" a man asks one day.

"What does this thing do?" asks a very short man in T-shirt and blue suspenders, looking the baby stroller up and down.

"Are they registered?" a woman asks.

"Are they big for their size?" asks a woman with a yipping dog in her handbag.

"Where are you going?" a man asks, swiveling his head around to survey the town, as though my presence at this particular longitude and latitude makes little sense.

"Do you think I could freeze my eggs?" asks a woman who looks too old to be worrying about it.

"You should be more careful," an older woman says, with disapproval.

· · ·

One day, a long time from now, when the babies are ten months old, Asher and I will take them for a walk. It will be a warm Saturday in November, one of those global-warming days, and Bronxville will be filled with people escaping the winter blues.

For the first time ever, Hannah and Barak will ride in the double-umbrella stroller and Jared will ride up high on my back, in one of Asher's old backpacks.

Asher will help me push the umbrella stroller through town. The five of us will promenade as usual, but something will strike me as different, odd, unbalanced.

We will make our usual circuit of Starbucks, video store, bagel store, organic food store, and then the supermarket. The weird feeling will nag at me. Something will feel wrong.

After forty-five minutes or so, I will realize what is out of kilter: not one person stops to comment about the babies.

Is my mathematical model for meeting the local population finally coming true? Or is it the absence of the visually dramatic baby carriage? Are the babies no longer an obvious curiosity because they are not displayed three in a row? Was their former popularity purely a result of clever packaging?

The babies will be older and their maturity will raise the possibility they are not triplets but three separate kids, cousins, siblings of different ages, even friends.

No immediate answer will come as Asher and I enjoy the unusual freedom of parading unnoticed through our morning routine, but after an hour or so I will feel that twinge of disappointment, like an aging movie star who finds, for the first time in his life, that no one recognizes him anymore.

NINE

Nature vs. Ferber

Jared looks so small and plump and pale when I unwrap his clothing and gently place him on the examining table in his powder blue onesie. I lean over and press my body against his to keep him warm and calm and still enough for the exam. He starts bawling when the urologist gently touches the ultrasound wand on his back. After a hundred ultrasounds of Roni to show us Jared, now we must look inside Jared. The babies are three and a half months old now.

The test is wrapped up in a few minutes. I wait for the results, dress Jared and hug him and congratulate him on what a trooper he is. The pediatric urologist, Dr. Poppas, sits down with us, as warm and gentle as any mom and more handsome than any movie star. I am not into Eastern religion, but Dr. Poppas has the most visible aura of pure goodness I have ever seen in an adult male. He says the enlargement in Jared's right kidney seems to be slowly shrinking. We need another ultrasound in six months, but

Dr. Poppas believes the problem is resolving itself as he hoped when he saw Jared at four weeks. I take a deep breath, and when I exhale, twelve months' worth of anxiety—a bellyful of acidic, noxious fumes—pours out of me. The nurses tickle Jared's feet and say he looks just like me.

At fifteen weeks now, Jared, biggest at birth, is still the largest, with chubby cheeks like mine that turn Pinocchio red when he feeds or laughs or cries. He knocks back an eight-ounce bottle easily now. Up until a few weeks ago, when Jared sat in the bouncy seat, he seemed distracted and could not focus quickly on visual stimuli. This led Ima and Roni to worry if he was a little slow. Roni snapped her fingers behind Jared's head and whistled at him to check his hearing.

Now that Jared is as alert and responsive as Barak and Hannah, the issue is put to rest, but this bizarre role reversal contradicted the natural family order, in which my mom and I played the official family worriers and Roni and her mother acted as principal harrumphers. I explain to Roni that our marriage rests on certain basic assumptions, chief among them that I will worry about the millions of minor problems that may befall the babies, the house, our finances, and our relationship, which she will firmly but tactfully lay to rest. Roni is empowered to agonize over the great, sweeping forces in our lives, releasing me to assume the role of cosmic comforter.

"What would happen if you gave Asher extra treats?" I say. "Our whole system would break down."

"Maybe you would stop giving him treats," Roni says. It's an intriguing theory. What happens if the neat one starts leaving socks and towels on the floor and drinks from the orange juice container? Would the messy one take offense and switch roles, or would the whole marriage spin down into the bottomless hole of negative synchronicity?

Jared is the most sensitive baby. Loud noises trigger a terrified startle reflex. When the three babies sit in their bouncy seats and the doorbell rings, Jared's arms and legs shoot out in all directions and he begins bawling, while the other two turn curiously to the sound. Jared cries the most often and requires the most consolation time. At night I walk around with Jared twice as much as Hannah and Barak combined.

One of the weirdest aspects of raising a baby girl is the automatic evaluation of her attractiveness. Friends and family comment about Jared and Barak's facial features, resemblance to other family members, personality quirks, even speculate about future career paths, but with Hannah every comment concerns her relative beauty. This is not flattering but annoying, because this is clearly untrue. Hannah has a square face and the bulging Stockler eyes of my father and his father, my grandfather Herbert, the trademarked bulging eyes that stare back at me from a faded 1922 portrait of taciturn Gittel Stockler, a paternal-family matriarch.

Every parent believes their daughter is beautiful, but, with four kids and some experience, I see Hannah is not. When strangers say how beautiful Hannah is, my reaction is to think they are simpleminded or short of conversation.

But why do I care if people think Hannah is beautiful— even if they are lying to be polite? Why do I so adamantly believe she is not? I haven't been able to admit this to Roni, because it would infuriate her, but now that Hannah's reflux is resolved I worry the least about Hannah. When the three babies are crying I pick up Hannah last and try to put her down first. Jared gets the most attention and Barak lands in the middle.

It is a natural flaw of parenting to empathize with one child more than another, and to rotate that prejudice over the years, deep within the irrational wilds of the heart, but it makes me feel terribly guilty. Of course, I am the guilty type and feel responsible when it rains. But I wonder why I am not bonding with Hannah. Is some of this unresolved hostility toward my father, whom she was born so closely resembling? Or—it gives me irritable bowel syndrome even to think it—does Hannah remind me of Roni, and have I tapped into a strange and unexplored well of resentment? As if our marriage isn't fractious enough.

One day when I am packing up the babies for a trip into town, Roni says, out of the blue, "Do you pay as much attention to Hannah as the boys?"

I am frozen with fear. The three kids have their bottles and toys lined up—what could she be talking about? Roni can't point to anything specific, but she worries I am not paying enough attention to our baby girl. If I don't pay enough attention to Hannah, she will have a lousy love life and date the wrong men and end up divorced and angry and a compulsive eater who wears nylon jogging suits day and night. Roni may be wacky but is rarely neurotic, and this blast of anxiety is like a tropical hurricane sneaking up on Florida without warning. I lie and say Hannah and I are doing fine.

At three and a half to four months, Hannah thankfully begins to lose the eerie Stockler bug-eyed trait. In fact, time and the loss of baby fat accentuates Hannah's beautiful blue-gray eye color, passed down from Roni's father, a fact that Roni's family seizes on desperately after years of hearing how Asher looks exactly like me.

The one real problem with Hannah is her volcanic temper, which shocks even Roni. If Hannah is hungry, wet, or not picked up with sufficient hustle, she will scream the paint off the ceiling. Each baby has his or her individual scream fingerprint, but Hannah hits the purest note of rage. And yet Hannah is the best sleeper of all the babies. At three months she begins to sleep for six hours at a stretch.

Barak is long and thin but growing quickly. He is the most sweet natured and pliable baby, infinitely patient and always willing to wait for his bottle or a clean diaper or removal from his crib. We rely on Barak for a short break in the daily chaos.

Once or twice a day the babies simultaneously fall into a fit of hysteria, their screams driving one another to greater heights of fury. If I am alone with them, I will laugh nervously at this debilitating storm of noise and try to lull them back down or separate them or distract them. I lack the emotional detachment to step back and let them exhaust themselves. The sound cuts through me, rendering me helpless, even though I know that in five or ten minutes a startling and alien quiet will once again descend.

So Barak is our little safety valve, and we treasure him for his complicity. Barak is starting to suck his thumb now, another sign of a child who holds his own. Barak still takes the longest to feed and often falls asleep during feedings with his pouty lower lip stuck out, trembling with drops of milk. We tease him about being lazy. Barak has wispy blond hair starting on top, like my brother, Paul. In fact, the shape of Barak's long face reminds me more and more of my brother Paul, especially as he grows older.

At night Barak is the wild card. Two or three nights in a row he will sleep soundly, but the next he wakes frequently with gas, a wet diaper, hacking coughs, loose bowel movements or the mystery crying, that awful, undecipherable unhappiness that tears out my heart while generating fantasies of sleeping on the beach in the Florida Keys.

Jared has become the real problem at night. By four months he begins to wake up once, twice, sometimes three or four times a night, crying inconsolably. Bottle, diaper, baby blanket, nothing soothes him, except when I take him out of his crib and walk around with him on my shoulder, moving continuously.

I create two baby-walking circuits to manage nighttime crying. The short circuit is one lap around the baby room with a turnaround in the hallway. The long version is out into the hallway, down to the bathroom, through Asher's bedroom, a few laps in the hallway, then back into the babies' room for a victory lap and a carefully calibrated slide off my arm, over the railing, and down into the pillowy caress of the crib.

Jared prefers the long circuit and demands that I hold him in a highly specific way—his body tucked into my chest, head resting on my shoulder, rear end and feet firmly supported. If his feet dangle loosely, he cries. If his head lolls about, he cries. And, most of all, if I stop moving or sit down, he cries. Sometimes I sit down in the rocking chair out of exhaustion and Jared begins crying instantly.

"Why can't I sit down? Why can't we sit down together for one minute?" I say.

How can a small baby be so sensitive to his relative position in the X, Y, and Z axes of 3-D space? Do babies have advanced gyroscopic sensitivities of which I am unaware? Can it be simple coincidence that the one activity that soothes him the most—walking around—is the most time-consuming and tiring solution?

I am too busy adjusting the minutiae of my Jared-soothing ritual to notice the bigger picture, which Roni coldly lays out one night after I loop into the master bedroom, where she is up late, watching TV.

I carefully slide Jared into the big bed, hoping this rare entry into its magical, mystical realms will soothe his angry heart, but Jared immediately begins crying and kicking. Jared senses his shift in 3-D space and the emergency bells clang. Jared demands to be returned to a position equal to a plumb line.

"You have to stop picking him up," Roni says.

Roni has no interest in my theory about Jared's spatial sensitivities. She feels my attempts to train the babies to sleep through the night have not only failed but have been subverted completely, and that it is Jared who is training me to bear him around.

"Imagine John Wayne carrying his horse around," Roni says. This is an old dispute—I am too lenient and unwilling to impart discipline. I jump through the babies' hoops and leave her to make and enforce the rules. If Jared isn't wet and doesn't need a bottle, we should let him cry and learn to calm himself down, Roni says, handing me our dog-eared but wholly ignored copy of *Solve Your Child's Sleep*

Problems, the classic baby-training text by Richard Ferber.

After several exhausting discussions that lead nowhere in arabesque circles, I consent to try and Ferberize Jared, even though I failed to Ferberize Asher.

"Asher Ferberized you," Roni says. I would sit with Asher at night, holding the fingers of his right hand tightly as he sucked on two fingers of his left hand, and wait until he fell asleep. I omit the fact that I loved sitting with Asher at bedtime and take the bullet for failing to train him instead.

While sleep deprived and fuzzy headed, I try to rebuild my daily schedule. First, I make peace with Nicky, devising projects to win new readers. I tell Nicky that while my travel schedule will be limited this year, I will start to travel by early next year. Nicky likes my ideas for expanding our readership and appears willing to live with my travel plans, although he insists we draw up a monthly travel schedule. Any jobs I interview for are trade magazine jobs in less appealing industries, like convention and tourism management. To make a career change now will require a massive effort and a cut in salary. But more instability and less income is not what I need now, so I postpone the job-changing issue for at least a year.

And so I try Ferber again, letting Jared cry for a few minutes longer every night. But for me, trying to ignore a crying baby is like trying to ignore a ringing doorbell. Hello? Hello!! What kind of lunatic pretends not to be home? I am here, here I am, at home, deep in the bosom of my son's caterwauling, pretending I am somewhere, and someone, else.

By the third night, when we reach ten minutes of waiting time, an angry voice rings out inside my skull. How
long will this noise continue? Why does it cut through my
head like a chainsaw? How long can this person scream?
Hours? Years?

After fifteen minutes of Jared's tirade, Barak wakes up,
unhappy and disoriented. I put both babies on my shoulder
and walk down the hallway with surround-sound crying,
closing the door to avoid waking Hannah. If Hannah wakes
up I don't know what I will do. With two babies on my
chest, I am in imminent danger of being outnumbered, not
a good situation, tactically. If Hannah wakes up I will have
to carry her in my teeth by the fabric of her onesie. If Asher
wakes up or the phone rings or I have to urinate, my op-
tions are depleted, and I will be a plane circling an airport
with no landing gear.

I stand at the door to our bedroom and watch Roni sleep
soundly, office work spread around her, TV and lights on.
I consider accidentally bumping into her, but she has
inched across to the far side of the bed into my territory.
Consciously or not, she has anticipated my cowardly strategy.

"Daddy!" I hear, from Asher's room.

"What?" I say.

"The babies are bothering me!" Asher says. "They're going to wake me up."

I'm not sure what to say. Asher talks in his sleep, not
just gibberish but grammatically correct sentences. I wait
outside his room, rocking the babies up and back.

"Pick me up," Asher says.

"I can't," I say. "I'm holding Jared and Barak."

"I can go on your shoulders," Asher says, ever the helpful

strategist. Like his mom, he always finds an angle. I will sit with him on his bed once the babies are in their cribs.

"Well, then, do you know where my Rugrats pen is?" Asher asks.

The Rugrats pen. It is 2:30 in the morning, I am standing in the hallway, at the top of the stairs, with two crying babies, and now I must solve the fate of the Rugrats pen. I mentally retrace the last time I saw the Rugrats pen, consider all the possible missing-Rugrats-pen scenarios. I wonder what my life will be like when I am up in the middle of the night searching for four Rugrats pens.

In about fifteen minutes I return Barak to his crib. Jared requires another fifteen minutes of my time, as if he resents sharing the real estate of my chest with Barak.

I don't see Roni the next morning. Later she e-mails me some passages from Ferber. When Roni wraps her mind around an idea, she finds it difficult to let go. Her passion for pursuing an argument sometimes outgrows the moral weight of the actual dispute. For example, she will agitate for years over selecting the color of fabric for a couch reupholstery job, but might decide we should all move to northern California and grow grapes after reading one article about grape-growing yuppie dropouts. "You said you wanted a woman who defies all clichés," she says, when I point this out.

I'm more a Penelope Leach person, overprotective, indulgent, love-them-first-and-set-them-straight-later. Roni is closer to Ferber—train them, change their behavior, improve them, mold them now, for their good and your own and the long-term health of the nation-state. There are loud, obnoxious children screaming away in every super-market in the land to prove her point. Leaches marry Ferbers all the time, but, like midwestern Lutherans who marry Methodists, it works as long as you don't quote chapter and verse at each other.

I agree to try one more time. I can't spend the next eighteen months walking across the hallway in the middle of the night, a zombie dad wandering through the graveyard of his own lost sleep.

Tonight I am exhausted—some nights are just worse than others. At about 1:00 A.M., I pace in the hallway with Jared after his fifteen Ferber minutes, but he isn't following the game plan and calming down. I deploy all my tricks, including the emergency football carry and my patented waddle walk, but he will not settle down.

"Shhh!" I beg. "Come on, I can't walk all night long. Please go back to sleep."

"If you let him cry, he'll eventually fall back to sleep," Roni says. "Crying makes them tired."

But what if this basic assumption is wrong? What if crying releases endorphins, like jogging, and only increases his energy level? What if crying is like training for the marathon and we are unwittingly creating our own Kenyan crying superstar?

I'm following the program, I say. "Barak and Hannah are going to start crying all the time," Roni says. "They'll be old enough in a month or two to realize Jared's getting more attention."

Jared needs to give me a break and now Roni is on my case. I still have the laundry, garbage, dishwasher, car, and the lights. The lights in the basement are on—

Jared's head pops off my shoulder. He is crying louder

now. Why is he crying louder? He is moving in the wrong behavioral direction. Jared has my full attention. He's been fed, changed, burped, mollycoddled. Jared starts twisting his head around and down, trying to pull away from me with lizardlike agility. I put him in the big bed next to Roni. She kisses him and hugs him and hands him back in exactly the same state of agitation. I try to shush him. I don't want to wake Barak.

Jared cries harder. I walk downstairs to the living room and around the kitchen and look at this beautiful bag of Cheese Doodles with their nutrient-rich orange flavoring and over here a pot charred with tomato sauce and onions and here's a black slab that might be a piece of a toy or possibly a hacked-up piece of decaying meat and the clock is ticking tick-tock on the wall and I see the moon through that window with the jelly fingerprints on it and look at this stack of unopened mail which may or may not have a friendly letter from the people at the car finance company whom we love to talk to oh so much and back we go up the stairs stepping over Mommy's underwear that Daddy forgot to wash and we are listening to Mommy snore now go Mommy go and do that sleepytime thing and look here's your crib all warm and snuggly soft. But the walking faster and talking has not helped. Jared is standing pat, fighting, crying louder. I am at least one long hour away from sleep. That's 2:30, then back up at 6:00, with luck.

"Please," I beg Jared. "Please stop crying!"

Jared cries louder. He jerks his head away from me. His face and neck muscles are red from exertion.

"Will you please shut up!" I yell, holding Jared out in front of me.

One pure moment of silence follows, clear and pure as

glacial runoff, and my heart sinks. Then Jared bursts out into pitiable, fearful wailing, fat tears dropping from his eyes like overripe apples in an orchard.

"I can't believe you yelled at him," Roni moans, from the bedroom.

I can't believe it either. Up until this point, I rarely yelled at Asher. My vision of fatherhood is organized around two guiding principles—to be home with my kids and to not yell at them, to be the opposite of my father, a nervous, high-strung, workaholic, self-centered dad who was never home and, when he was around, was prone to scream at my brother and me for disturbing him in his darkroom or his workroom or whatever brilliant creative activity he chose to occupy himself with. The not-yelling father is crucial to my self-esteem and is essential to my identity.

I hug Jared tightly as he riots in my arms and tell him how sorry I am, how much I love him, what a bad father I am, what a wonderful little bald-headed squeezably chunkalicious stinky-pot of a nudgemacker he is and how I am going to buy him a puppy and teach him to catch a baseball and lie with him in fields of tall grass, staring up at the drifting clouds, provided we are covered by the proper antitick medication. I berate myself for this outburst. Jared is only a baby and it doesn't matter how tired I am. He needs me to be his rock, even when I feel like loose gravel.

After a few minutes Jared reaches the peak of his panic and eases down the other side. The lull in his wailing allows me to hear the cries coming from the baby room. Hannah and Barak are awake now.

Roni lumbers into the hallway, blinking and rubbing her face. She sees how angry I am at myself for losing my temper and gives me a supportive rub on the back. It means a lot in this moment. Thankfully, she does not attempt to take Jared and comfort him, one of those husband-wife moves that seems helpful but is subversively critical.

"Daddy!" Asher yells. "The babies are bothering me. I have to go to school tomorrow!"

"*Shhhh!*" I say. "I really need everyone to stop screaming. Please?"

Roni leans back at the wall and smiles at me in a way I have never seen before, probably, I realize later, the way I would look if I watched her handle a stressful situation in her office.

The next morning I put the Ferber book down in the basement in the same corner with the untouched bag of pacifiers, the box of stuffed animals we never put in their room to cut down on house dust, and the annoyingly cute, full-body Halloween costumes we never made them wear.

TEN

The Movable House, the Lemon Cookies, and Being Crushed: My Wife

Fatherhood is easy. Marriage is hard.

Kids need love, attention, and patience. Wives need all of that, plus ESP. If you don't know your wife has been yearning for that cement dog statue she saw in a Connecticut salvage yard six months ago, and you buy her a lovely yet not ostentatious string of natural pearls for her birthday instead, without checking with her best friend Marla in advance, your failure will be absolute, inexcusable, and irredeemable. Trying to read a wife's mind is like trying to look two minutes into the future. It sounds easy but is quite impossible.

Roni wakes me up at 2:00 in the morning.

"Are you sleeping?" she says.

"No?" I say.

"I have an idea," Roni says.

During the day, when I could hide behind a couch or

invent a chore in the basement, this kind of announcement is alarming enough. But now, in the dead of night, I curl up in a ball and try to let the horror wash over me. I breathe slowly. There is nothing I can do. Resistance is futile.

"Chocolate broccoli," she says, miming with her hands the packaging for a candy bar. "Chocco-brocco."

She turns to see my reaction.

"I like it," I say. "I'll make some phone calls?"

She puts her leg over mine and falls back to sleep. It could have gone the other way—way, way, way the other way.

My wife is weird. I have a weird wife. I could say Roni does everything in life the hard way, in the naive belief that the world will bend around her singular vision, but that would be judgmental. To her mind the world is just a vast and illogical sphere that could benefit from her benevolent tweaking.

Consider the movable house. After living in the rented house in Bronxville for several months, we start to maybe possibly theoretically conjecturally consider when we might take a few steps toward buying a house. The prices for houses in commuting distance to New York City are astronomical, absurd. An unrenovated four-bedroom cookie-cutter Colonial from the 1970s on a quarter-acre lot might cost $400,000 to $1.5 million or more, depending on the town and the street. One night Roni discovers, on a Web site, some beautiful Victorian houses situated in small towns in Upstate New York. The houses are selling for $50,000, $60,000, maybe $80,000, less than a good master bathroom renovation would cost in the New York suburbs.

"I have an idea," Roni says, calling from work one afternoon.

"I hear something beeping—" I say.

"—and we can move this house I found down here on a boat, and buy a piece of land for it," she jumps in. "It will cost a lot less than building a new house."

Somehow, somewhere, Roni read about entire houses being pried up off their foundations and moved with cranes and hydraulic jacks and river barges and trucks. I point out that the closest river is the Bronx River, which is as wide as our dinner table, but she does not consider this discouraging. We are close to the mighty Hudson River, and if she has not seen a single-family house floating down the Hudson River one sunny afternoon, on the way to its new home, she can easily imagine it.

She spends two months investigating house-moving operations. She speaks to engineering firms, calls real estate brokers for vacant lot prices, and analyzes the insurance risks. It's not that her idea is so ludicrous, once you get past the peculiar grandiosity of it. If we paid $75,000 for the four-bedroom house, $100,000 to move it, and $250,000 for the lot, that would be a total investment of about $425,000, about $100,000 to $200,000 less than the average four-bedroom in our area. Of course, that's on paper, and many ideas look great on paper, but do not necessarily translate into good homes in the physical world. Eventually the plan runs out of steam or loses out to entropy.

· · ·

When we were newlyweds, living near Columbia University on the Upper Upper West Side of Manhattan, Roni developed a craving for lemon cookies. Not just any lemon cookies, rare enough to begin with, but a very specific lemon cookie. A thin lemon cookie, not too sweet, with no frosting on top or cream inside.

Roni had eaten these lemon cookies for many years; they were quite popular; she was not sure of the brand; she couldn't remember the last time she had eaten them, or where she bought them; and could I please go buy her some?

I scurried off to the Columbia University supermarket, but had no luck. I walked through all the bodegas, fruit and vegetable shops and gourmet stores in the fifteen blocks closest to our apartment. To return empty-handed from a strictly itemized shopping expedition would invite charges of male incompetence—real or feigned—so I brought home five or six cookie variations most closely matching her description, even though only one of them contained any lemon and only one was remotely thin.

Roni was very upset. These pitiful imposters were an insult to cookie eaters everywhere. My failure only intensified her inexplicable craving.

Days of lemon cookie pursuit crumbled into weeks. I toured Manhattan's largest supermarkets, prowled the most expensive gourmet shops, haunted the oddest corner stores, interrogating managers, bakers, truckers, and store owners. I scoured Yellow Pages and food magazines. Every night, when Roni came home late from work, tired and beaten down, she would look at me with those sad where-are-my-lemon-cookie eyes.

Where are the lemon cookies, the lemon cookies? I say

to myself as I ride the Number Three train to Penn Station. When I go to the laundry room I wonder where could the lemon cookies be? When I read a book, magazine, or newspaper, and I stumble across the accursed word *lemon*, my blood pressure skyrockets.

One day I eat lunch in a diner with my friend, Michael Billig, and recount the lemon cookie ordeal. A nearby waitress jumps into the conversation. She knows about these lemon cookies. She loves the lemon cookies. She ate them all the time.

My heart races as I calculate how much of a tip I can leave a waitress from a foreign station. I drift back into reality with a sinking feeling in my stomach.

The company stopped making the lemon cookies about twenty years ago and is long out of business. Of this she is quite confident. In a few days I confirm this story with an old-timer at a small bakery in the West Village.

"That can't be," Roni says. "I just had them a little while ago . . ."

Roni looks at me like a dog abandoned by the side of the road. What am I supposed to say? That when she looks for lemon cookies, the universe will rearrange itself? A black hole will open and plunge me back into a time and place more conducive to lemon cookie acquisition?

She looks at me sadly for a few moments, changes the channel on the TV, and that is the end of that. Roni has bizarre and demanding tastes, but she doesn't waste time feeling sorry for herself.

Our life together has always been odd. After we met through the personal ads, seven full weeks passed before

we decided we disliked each other little enough to float
the trial balloon of a kiss. Then Roni went off to Czecho-
slovakia for two weeks with her girlfriend Nancy, who lived
across the hall. Roni and Nancy tiptoed back and forth
across the hallway with gossip and casseroles and clipped-
out magazine articles, like college girls, and fought constantly. Nancy was on my side, having decided I was good
medicine for Roni. I always did well with girlfriends and
their mothers, which, I discovered later, is counterproductive, and only works when the woman wants to get married.

This kind of insanity continued for eight or nine months.
After seven or eight months, Roni and I became engaged,
although neither one of us actually asked the question. We
both accused the other of intimating that we should probably get married, in the most cowardly way imaginable, and
then argued about whose fault it was that nothing had been
said directly, and we didn't have a proper engagement, like
people in *The New York Times* style section, or the movies,
until my mom became so exasperated by the sheer incompetence of the whole situation that she drove up to the city
in a cloud of Parliament smoke and stuck an engagement ring
into my hand that had been in her family for generations.

"You know what to do with this, I hope," said my mother.

"It's not edible, right?" I said.

"You're not still taking the subways, are you?" said my
Mom. She worried about me living in the city, even after
ten years.

"Only when I have to buy heroin downtown," I said.

I'm sure my mom expected her ring to be lost down a
drain or mixed up in a garbage bag, and I don't think she
was too crazy about me marrying anyone, especially Roni,

whom one could peg as difficult from fifty yards away, but my mother was very sweet and supportive and made sure I put the ring away in a safe place before she left. My mom married a quirky, brilliant, high-maintenance man who turned out to be a self-centered husband, and I could tell she was disappointed I hadn't picked a traditional, warm, loving Jewish girl, but she never said a word about it, except to say she only wanted me to be happy, a kind of universal maternal coded message that I could interpret any which way, depending on the situation. But I knew exactly what she meant.

For years, whenever I reacted to Roni with anger or frustration, not understanding how I could have married someone whose brain could attack a problem and calculate a solution so opposite and counterintuitive to mine, Roni always shot back the same annoying answer: "You said you wanted a woman who *defies all clichés*."

"A woman who defies all clichés" was the line from my personal ad, which Roni saved as a keepsake (or as evidence to use against me). You need to be careful what you wish for, especially if you're foolish enough to commit it to print.

I moved from my illegal East Side sublet into the construction zone Roni referred to as home, near Columbia University. Roni's apartment had no working kitchen, the walls and ceilings were half Sheetrocked and huge chunks of plaster and mortar squatted on couches and chairs, as if they lived there. One day I was looking for ketchup in the bombed-out shell of the kitchen and found a fully operational jackhammer.

Roni was close friends with a fiftyish man named Bob who had a grown daughter living in Mexico. Bob was a journeyman kind of guy—he worked on construction crews and on TV commercial crews, he did odd jobs for building supers, he sold Mexican fruit, he wrote short stories. Bob was very sweet and gentle and kind, like Mr. Rogers, but extremely smart and well read. Bob was Roni's construction guru and coincidentally best friends with one of the men Roni stopped dating to make room for me. At first I didn't know whether Bob was making circuitous conversation or keeping me under surveillance.

As a home renovator, Bob was a crazed perfectionist who would take a year to finish painting a plain old twelve-by-ten bedroom because he kept getting distracted and starting new, tangentially related projects, which begat still other projects, until one day he'd be buying plaster gargoyles at a salvage yard in Delaware that had something to do with a roof garden that existed as a sketch on a long lost napkin.

Bob was a serial project digresser, an especially wicked trait combined with Roni's tendency to be a serial project abandoner. Instead of finishing the closets in the master bedroom, Roni and Bob would begin new projects in the kitchen, den, living room and hallway, each inching forward mysteriously. Roni should have married Bob, who treated Roni with gentle, puppylike devotion, and if Bob were a little younger this might have been a book about dating problems after forty.

Roni hated anything related to water—swimming, boating, the ocean, beach vacations, lakes, and rivers. She did not drink water or use ice. She did not care for anything watery—hot or iced tea, coffee, frozen drinks, ice, snowballs, skiing. She hated action movies, zoos, college and professional sports, chopped meats, modern furniture, any rock music after 1968 (except for the Beatles), David Letterman, and pineapple. She ate only dark, unsweetened chocolate. She considered veal disgusting because of the way it was raised, but she loved foie gras. Most of her casual clothes were vintage, bought in thrift stores, with a special predilection for black crushed velvet. She had trouble falling asleep and would stay in bed until 12:00 or 1:00 P.M. on a Saturday afternoon if you didn't wake her.

Roni loved to be pressed down by a crushing, heavy weight while relaxing or trying to fall asleep. She begged me to buy her a king-size bedspread lined with lead. "Like the lead blanket you wear when you have an X ray taken," Roni said. When she couldn't sleep, she made me lie down on top of her, all 230 pounds, torso to torso, arms to arms, legs to legs, crushing her down into the mattress like in the cartoons when the Coyote was crushed into the desert floor.

"Are you still breathing?" I would say, looking down. "I can't tell."

Roni didn't open her mail for months at a time. She mixed up music and movie references from different decades like cultural cole slaw. She never heard of Brian DePalma, U2, Roberto Clemente, Dan Aykroyd, or postmodern fiction. She missed the second half of the '70s and most of the '80s. She loved Nat King Cole, the Drifters, *All My Children* and any TV mystery, the more British or obscure, the better.

Roni was nothing like the woman I imagined I would marry. I saw myself with a dark-haired, exotic, intellectual, artistic type. Roni was a short, red-haired, type A corporate attorney by day and an iconoclast by night. She arrived at our first date wearing construction boots and a faded T-shirt from the Omega Institute, a hippie-dippie, New Age retreat in Upstate New York, where, coincidentally, I once spent a weekend with my ex-girlfriend Dina, who was dark-haired, intellectual, exotic, and mysterious. After our breakup, Dina and I remained close friends and Roni was as naturally suspicious of her as I was of Roni's most recent ex. Years later I realized that, under different circumstances, Roni and Dina might have been great friends.

Facing the flaws you see in yourself is not nearly as difficult as facing the flaws others point out. After six years of marriage, I have to admit that many of Roni's criticisms of me are true. The man who brought her flowers and found her every word fascinating and who listened to her problems and schemes and ideas for hours with a loving twinkle in his eye is not the man who is laughing out loud at SpongeBob SquarePants in the TV room with a sixty-four-ounce bottle of Fresca in his lap. The man who braved ballroom dancing lessons and spent weeks planning romantic bed-and-breakfast getaways is no more. The man who watched every bite of food he put in his mouth and ran up and down the stairs in his building seven days a week is long gone, replaced by a tired-eyed man forty pounds heavier. She lost Doting Man and found herself married to Daddy Man. When she complains I love the kids more than her, and that the marriage books say a husband must put his wife's needs first, I cringe. Comparing types of love is like comparing apples and oranges, but, even though she is wrong, she is right. The daddy part of me is more perfectly synchronized than the husband part. I don't know exactly how or why it happened, and the only thing I can do is conjure up some of that old playfulness and infatuation and magic. It's still there when I see her gardening with three mud-covered kids, or singing to the Supremes in the car, or wandering off in a department store with a lopsided grin on her face, or wearing that faded powder blue cable sweater in which she looks like the kooky girl I first dated. The love gets buried alive under the to-do lists, the squabbling, the power struggles, and the money anxiety.

Roni and I bicker over meaningless things. We agree it is a waste of time. Sometimes we are in the middle of an argument about what Asher should be eating, and then we will segue into a fight about who started the argument, who apologized for the last argument, and then we will transition into increasingly digressive arguments, and in another hour we will be sulking, silently, both mystified as to how we got here.

For a while I believed Roni engineered these fights as a weird kind of alternative entertainment. This theory dates back to the renovation of Roni's apartment. One day she sent me to the local hardware store to buy an eighth-inch, round-top wood screw. But the store only had eighth-inch, flat-top wood screws or three-sixteenth-inch, round-top wood screws. Whichever way I prioritized the components of the screw—size, wood versus metal, type of head—this was inevitably the worst choice.

"I can use a bigger screw, but I can't have the head sticking up!" Roni would say, pointing to a gaping hole in the wall, where something indeterminate was about to go wrong thanks to my screwhead-selection ignorance. Back to the store I went. The next time, however, when I applied the head-style criteria, and bought the wrong size, right head, screw, I found that screw size was the most important criterion.

One day I bought four or five of the closest screw types, but this foolproof plan backfired when she got angry at my lack of understanding the job at hand. When I told her this was lemon-cookie karma working itself out and that she was purposely sending me on doomed missions, she shrugged me off. Eventually we laughed every time she sent me out the door, both of us anxious to find out exactly how the enterprise would self-destruct.

But now when we argue about chores that fail miserably and how we waste our precious time, Roni will say, "You used to tease me about this." I remind her she used to think I was funny.

I should try to appreciate Roni more instead of agitating over all the weirdness. I should let things slide. I shouldn't argue back. I should let her say her piece and just be quiet.

These are the words I repeat as I look over the crowd of moms at the birthday party in Asher's nursery school gymnasium. Asher has started nursery school in Scarsdale, the upscale suburb a few towns north of Bronxville, because the school day here continues until 6:30, which gives me enough time to hoof it home from the city.

The three- and four-year-old kids run around under the watchful eye of Coach Ricky and the moms in their Chanel suits and museum-quality faded jeans and $600 Jimmy Choo boots, who fuss and swoon and schedule play dates into the twenty-second century. Suburban moms schedule play dates with the intensity that Stalin shuffled around his ministries.

Then there is Roni, huddling with the janitor, asking questions about the buffing pads on the floor waxing machine for some future, vaguely defined, home renovation project. I talk to the other moms about car pools and summer camp plans.

Out here in the suburbs, people see us raising triplets, and a fourth, plus mom is a high-powered attorney, dad is a writer and Mr. Mom type, and they wonder. The moms stay home and run the systems while the dads work on Wall Street or are partners at Manhattan law firms. If you own an antique store or a jewelry store passed down within your family, you are a radical. The conformist environment is like a thick plate of glass that magnifies our weirdness a hundredfold. Roni doesn't mix in with the moms and I only connect with the dads who hate their law firms and wish they could own a fishing boat—both of them.

But we were weird before the kids arrived. Now that we are a family of six, I feel the weirdness multiplying, and it makes me afraid, because I want my kids to be well adjusted and successful and fit in to everyday life in a way I never did.

Roni, however, is drifting in the opposite direction. Fitting in to suburban America isn't a priority for her at all. In fact, she considers fitting in a negative. She says we should move to a small town somewhere out in that mythological American landscape where people survive on less and don't buy into materialism, where we can grow our own vegetables, make our own clothes, bottle jellies and jams, and listen to the timber wolves sing at night. We could live in another country, learn new languages, travel by minivan.

"That was an Albert Brooks movie," I say. "It ended badly."

Roni doesn't want to fight the weirdness but open the door to it, let it wash over us, transform us and carry us away to our destiny.

I argue that we owe our kids the choices we never had. Roni spent her first ten years living with her mother, father, sister, and grandmother in a one-bedroom apartment. I grew up in a house with unpainted rooms, a mother who worked in a shoe store, a father who lost all our money in the stock market. Shouldn't we do better by them? Isn't that the American way?

We're not slaves to culture. Asher doesn't have a Game Boy or Nintendo, we don't own Stickley furniture, our house is a mess, we don't have a cleaning woman, and the triplets wear hand-me-downs with holes in them. Roni and I buy new clothes for ourselves once a year. We haven't spent money on a vacation since Roni was pregnant with Asher. The women who baby-sit our kids all own larger TV sets.

I want the kids to have choices. Let them apply to Harvard or Stanford or USC Film School. Let them study in an ashram or trek in Nepal before college. Let them explore their whims and enjoy the hands-on life-planning guidance we didn't. Roni and I come from lower-middle-class families who sacrificed everything, but didn't understand social connections. We went to state universities, worked our way through college, battled for jobs. Our families didn't know how to help us.

Roni's parents never socialized. But Roni doesn't equate weird with antisocial. She thinks we can be weird *and* social. Not here in the middle, not in the suburbs, I say.

But maybe that's the whole point. Maybe the lesson behind Roni's crazy house-moving scheme was that we should live somewhere else, somewhere normal, where you can buy a house for $250,000 and live on $50,000 a year.

A thousand small towns out there would have us. I have crisscrossed the country a dozen times. We could live in a college town like Oneonta, New York, or Madison, Wisconsin. We could live outside of Raleigh-Durham, North Carolina, or in Charlottesville, Virginia. We could try Doylestown, Pennsylvania, or one of the Amish towns in Lancaster County. In the Upper Peninsula of Michigan, one town after another is sparklingly beautiful and full of waitresses who call you "hon" and the blue-plate specials cost less than a large latte in New York City. I love the desert and would be happy outside Sedona, Arizona, or Santa Fe, New Mexico, somewhere outside the antique-store zone.

Roni is ready to pack up and move, but the one thing holding us back is family. Roni's parents, sister, niece and nephews are in Schenectady, New York. My mom and grandmother are in Langhorne, Pennsylvania, south of Trenton. The only other reason not to make a major leap is fear of the unknown, a trait I thought we shared equally.

But now I realize that Roni is ready to jump off the cliff and go, right now, just to see what happens next, leaving me to play the sad and thankless role of little old lady.

"Let's do it," Roni says. "Let's just pack up our stuff in the truck and go."

We've been through so much change already. I feel as if I am coming up for air in white foam, after being knocked down by a series of huge waves.

"The last time we moved, we needed a twenty-four-foot tractor trailer," I remind her.

"We'll sell it, give it all away," she says. "It's all junk."

Then why does she go to tag sales and buy more of it? I wonder, but I don't say it. Even old dogs learn new tricks once in a while.

Roni is itching for more adventure, as if the four kids were not adventure enough. She wants the kids to learn what a plumb line is, to bake bread from scratch, to spot tiger tracks, to recognize leaves and berries you can eat when you're lost.

"You should teach a class," I say. " 'What you never learned in college.' "

"Very funny," Roni says.

At 2:00 A.M. I am awakened by an elbow in my kidney.

"I have an idea," Roni says. After so many years of dreading these very words, and breaking out in a flop sweat, I fold my hands behind my head and say I am ready to listen. I am sure she can feel my smile cracking open the darkened bedroom.

"Okay," she says, setting the tone. "Gourmet box lunches for elementary school kids. . . ." I listen to her as she dances off into her idea, thinking, not bad, not bad. She has a lot more to give the world than another SEC filing. Maybe what we need is a husband, to bring home the six-figure income.

ELEVEN

Chaos Theory

The days pass like months, the months like days.

The babies are five months old now. The peach fuzz on Jared's bald head is filling in, a feminine face emerges from the putty of Hannah's baby fat, and Barak develops a crooked and mischievous smile.

With all the outside pressure on us, our marriage should be like a foxhole, but sometimes we're too busy bickering to mount a good defense. Roni deals with unfriendly and insulting clients, who sometimes bad-mouth her to her boss in childish internal power struggles. Her law firm is understaffed and she often works late just to wait for a word processor to open up.

At my office, our new parent company has told me to retool the magazine and create more how-to articles and white papers that explain the nuts and bolts of digital technologies, written by hardware and software manufacturers. The beauty of such stories is that they are supplied free— no annoying writers to pay. The stories also get us past drinks and dinner and right into bed with advertisers. The downside is that our subscribers are reading quasi-publicity materials disguised as journalism.

We are drowning in disorganization at home. Financially we are in disarray—trying to pay two baby-sitters, falling behind in our estimated quarterly tax payments to the IRS, our savings gone. Gorillas in zoos have a better credit rating than we do. Every two weeks I take a moving box full of unopened mail down to the basement out of sheer desperation.

We can't live in a falling-down rental house forever. But housing prices are rising 10 percent a year in Westchester County. The starter house we looked at two years ago in Katonah for $450,000 that had considerable flaws now lists for $625,000 and seems perfect and delightful in out-of-our-price-range retrospect.

I spent a lot of time in the Florida Keys when I was in my twenties. We could live down there. The kids would grow up fishing and swimming and learning how to pilot a skiff, and I could be the eccentric muckraking editor of the local newspaper, and Roni could grow herbs and make coral-encrusted gift boxes and collect driftwood. Aside from Roni's hatred of the water and my fear of hurricanes and melanomas and insects, it's an interesting plan.

One night I sit up late, watching the kids sleep, and wonder if we are cursed to scrape by and worry about money forever. You can't be a responsible parent without worrying about money, but every minute spent worrying about money is wasted and irretrievable.

· · ·

And then I wake up at 5:00 A.M., anxious because the house is too quiet. Something must be wrong! I sneak into the babies' room, careful not to touch the creaky door or bump into Barak's crib or trip over the toys. The creeping summer morning sun is filtering in through the blinds. I look down at the three cribs, arrayed in an L along two walls of the room. My two boys and my girl are sound asleep in their fuzzy polyester PJs. The little sighs and lip smacks and nose snorts and whimpers and farts and crib-kickings fill the air with blissful white noise and as they wake up and see me they smile and clap and call my name. I am overcome. I must have been Mahatma Gandhi or Joan of Arc or Moses' personal assistant in a previous life to collect a reward this bountiful. I take the babies out of their cribs and we roll around on the carpet in the crackling strips of sunlight.

Once a week an old man or woman stops me on the street as I push the babies around. They grab my arm, squeeze it surprisingly hard, lean in to me, and whisper, urgently, "You're a very rich man." When I look them in the eyes and tell them they are right, they seem utterly relieved to know that wisdom is not extinct yet in the world, that their cherished value system will not die out with them, despite the general evidence of foolishness and moral anarchy all around.

The babies are six months old now and Hannah is the first to hold her bottle. To feed them together, I sit the babies on the floor in their bouncy seats, prop pillows on their stomachs, and line bottles up on the pillows, the nipples tilted down into their mouths. I pogo around the room adjusting bottles and pillows and seats. Now I wrap Jared's and Barak's hands around their bottles and encourage them to copy their sister.

"Girls are smarter," Roni says. She is sitting on the floor, taking pictures of Hannah. She is thrilled that Hannah is holding her bottle first, because she knows how much competition Hannah will face over the years from her brothers. I take the camera and tell Roni to sit with Hannah in her lap. Roni moves around, adjusting her legs, and Roni instinctively holds out her hand to keep Hannah's bottle from falling, but we both look down at the same time to see Hannah clutching her bottle fiercely, emptying the bottle with happy, noisy grunts. Roni looks up at me, and I know exactly what she is thinking—Hannah eats like a Stockler.

The boys each have two Sunday outfits. They look handsome, but slightly awkward, in button-down shirts, but Hannah looks like a whole different child in pink and taffeta and lace. Roni and I debate whether to nudge Hannah toward being a girly girl or to let her be one of the boys. Roni leans toward the girly girl approach, but my instinct is to let Hannah be a tough chick, so I won't have to spend so many sleepless nights in high school. I remind Roni that she wore work boots to our first date and her favorite birthday presents are power tools, and warn her not to transfer her unresolved femininity issues onto Hannah. Roni buys Hannah Barbie dolls, which she loves, but the ballerina dolls she dumps behind the couch. This is a good sign to me. Hannah's personality will flourish without parental engineering.

At seven months the babies all sit up straight, gurgle a few words, and hold their bottles. When they finish drinking, they wing the bottles over their heads like frat boys tossing out empties. Once in a while Jared beans me right on the head—he has the best arm—and they all crack up.

Asher becomes impatient with the pace of the growing-up process. "When will they be big enough to play with me?" he says. "What's taking so long?" Asher stands over the three babies as they giggle and laugh, waiting for something substantial to happen. If Asher is three, and the babies are seven months old, he has been waiting the equivalent of six middle-aged-person years, which must be frustrating.

Asher is spending the summer at a sports camp. He climbs on a little yellow school bus every morning with a bag lunch, swims laps in the Olympic-sized pool, plays soccer, and does arts and crafts. The first few days, I shadowed the bus to check up on the driver. Roni finds out and goes ballistic, so I neglect to mention my difficulty adjusting to the fact that Asher is old enough to spend the whole day away at camp.

Roni doesn't buy my theory that parents naturally divide into overprotection and autonomy camps. She thinks I spend too much time home with the kids and I am too soft with them and too indulgent and have been turned into a loving but indentured servant.

Barak and Hannah are packed into the umbrella stroller and Jared rides up in the backpack carrier. Jared grips the front of the backpack and his wide, bald head pokes out the top, like Kilroy. Asher helps push, putting his body in front of mine to hijack the job. Roni compares Jared to Asher, who also loved sitting up in the backpack and looking around. Roni says Asher and Jared look alike and I sense a special connection growing between the two boys.

But Asher instinctively knows not to favor any of the babies over the others. If he has a toy to show off, he carefully displays it to each one in turn, even changing the order the next time around. Asher amazes me with his emotional sensitivity. If I am downstairs and one of the babies starts crying in their room, I send Asher for a report, and receive a solid diagnosis most of the time. The only reason the system fails is when he torments them, which is still rare, although I suspect the protect/torment equation will change once the babies are old enough to rebel against his authority.

Asher is especially helpful at feeding time. The babies now sit in three modified high chairs, plastic baby seats with trays strapped onto dining room chairs. In the morning Asher pours Cheerios on the babies' trays. The babies love to eat and each one has a completely different style. Hannah takes two fists full of Cheerios and jams them into her mouth as fast as they will go. We warn her to slow down.

Jared picks at the Cheerios and fools around with them, looking to get a laugh—Cheerios on his head, Cheerios in the air, Cheerios on the floor.

Barak eats the Cheerios methodically, one after the other, his arm moving up and down like an oil derrick.

The babies quickly grow bored with the expensive organic baby food. When Asher digs into scrambled eggs or buttered bagel, the babies are so wide-eyed with hunger it would be heartless to deny them. They graduate quickly to Asher's diet—scrambled eggs, toast with crust cut off, bagel and butter, chicken nuggets, spaghetti with butter, crackers, and string cheese.

Lunch and dinner may take an unpredictable turn— three plates of spaghetti heaved across the room, chicken nugget pieces disappearing into nooks and crannies of the kitchen, milk spilled under ancient radiator covers—but we reach the maximum mayhem quotient less frequently than I expected. The babies have my genes and treat food with reverence.

Jared is the neatest eater. When he finishes his bagel, barely a trace of butter remains on his face and hands. He is instinctively fastidious and very unhappy if he spills something on his shirt.

Hannah is voracious. She eats until she or the food is removed. Hannah lives as though eating were a competition, which it will be, someday, because once the last piece of grilled chicken is gone, that will be that. Roni and I don't know if she is eating aggressively because of anxiety over future deprivation or because of my chow hound genes.

Barak is the messiest. After bread and butter his hair is as slick and shiny as a twenty-five-year-old stock broker. At night I find Cheerios tucked into the folds of his onesies from that morning and the juice stains on his shirts could be an homage to Jackson Pollock. But Barak takes great pleasure in eating, and if he revels in the untidiness of the act, more power to him. When he is happy I am happy. If the laundry basket is more than half his clothing casualties, he is simply a leader in his field.

.   .   .

It is the end of October and the babies are nine months old. They show no indication that they plan to walk any-time soon, even though Asher walked at nine months. Roni spends hours holding their hands and waltzing them across the floor, hooting and clapping and jumping up and down in encouragement. Hannah pulls herself across the floor on her rear end, backward, dragging her legs behind her. The boys crawl on all fours with crazy grins on their faces, gig-gling as they plow up and over obstacles. Sometimes the three babies pile up in the middle of the floor like a car wreck on the freeway. Peals of laughter follow as they re-alize the absurdity of their predicament and try to disen-tangle. A foot lands in a mouth or an elbow meets a chin and they fight like three wolverines dropped into a pit.

Their personalities are distinct. Jared is the most self-conscious—he is cute and he knows it—and works the room for attention. His brown hair is filling in thickly and he has a rakish little swirl falling down perfectly in the middle of his forehead. The baby fat is melting away to reveal an extremely handsome boy with the same knowing twinkle in his eye Asher had. But Jared is still the most easily insulted and injured; the slightest scratch causes him to yowl with paroxysms of pain. He still schemes the hard-est to have me pick him up and carry him around at all hours.

Hannah has a tousled mop of dark hair that doesn't want to settle down into anything resembling a hairstyle. She looks like she just hopped off the back of a speedboat. But she is developing a fierce independent streak and sets her jaw when unhappy in a way that leaves no doubts. She is the most diffident of the babies and in her tantrums remains emotionally unreachable. If someone takes her bottle away, she screams bloody murder until we cave in. You don't mess with Hannah.

Despite her fearsome temper, Hannah displays an amazing maternal side. One day Asher accidentally klonks Jared on the head with a toy, and when Jared starts bawling, Hannah crawls over and hugs him. We start calling her "the little mommy."

Barak is still the easiest one. He waits patiently for his bottle, never fussing as long as his yellow blanket is within reach. He sucks his thumb and not only enjoys it but considers it a funny habit for a creature his age. Barak falls sound asleep in every car ride, out cold before I finish backing the car out of the driveway. Barak has caught up with Jared in height and is growing the fastest. With his blond fuzzy hair and spray of freckles and runny nose he also seems the most fragile. He is the most prone to congestion and runny nose, and he coughs the most when the house is cold.

Jared's and Barak's first word is "Dada," which drives Roni crazy. Jared's and Barak's second word is "Asha," for Asher—they rhyme it with "pasha." The boys regard Asher with a bristling combination of awe, fear, and love. Mommy and Daddy are their lifelines, but Asher is at their level and omnipotent. Jared especially loves to say "Asha" and smiles with delight when he hears himself.

Jared wakes up the most at night, pulling himself up by the bars of the crib to cry "Dada." I hear the whole process—he rolls around in his crib, the springs squeak, he hoists himself up, and then there is a long pause as he realizes he is trapped in his crib when his big-shouldered, warm-blooded father waits only a few feet away. This seems a crime to him, to be only a few feet from the wide welcoming arms, yet cruelly abandoned in his squeaky old cage.

"Dada!" Jared yells. "Dada!"

"He *smells* you," Roni says. How else could he wake up from a deep sleep and know I have snuck in to replenish the tissue box? Is Roni insulting Jared or me?

A new phase in the nighttime games begins. Now that the babies can pull themselves up and deploy sensory techniques, my freedom of movement is severely restricted. I no longer can enter the room at night to put away folded laundry or change the diaper pail—a waking baby does not justify the task.

But I still change the babies' diapers at midnight, because Barak and Hannah will chafe if left all night in a wet diaper. Sometimes I walk into the room to retrieve lost keys or coagulating milk bottles or turn the radio down and hear Jared rustle. I might take refuge behind the closet door. I hear Jared's voice, "Dada," weak from sleep, then a stressful pause in the action, followed by the noise of him settling back down. If he catches me in the middle of the room I stop, drop and roll under one of the cribs, hiding from the searchlight of his awareness. The day he catches my leg or ass sticking out from under the crib all my maneuvers will be irretrievably compromised.

Rocky and Hannah's cribs are back to back against the hallway wall, and Jared's crib is alone against the outside wall of the house, so the window creates a buffer zone of about three open feet between the cribs. The foot of Jared's crib is normally draped with extra blankets that block his view, and sometimes I duck down in this space under the window. One night I am crouching down here as I hear Jared rustling, his subconscious mind weighing the rewards of wakefulness against REM sleep. Then I hear a voice.

"Dada?" the voice says. I turn my head and here is Hannah's little face, inches from mine.

"Shhhh," I say.

"Dada?" Hannah says. It must strike even a nine-month-old absurd to find her thirty-seven-year-old father crouching in the darkness beneath her crib.

"I don't want Jared to wake up," I whisper.

Hannah blinks at me, confused, then looks into Jared's crib. If she sees one hair of Jared I will have two crying babies. Instead, Hannah lays her head back down, sticks her tushie in the air, her thumb in her mouth, and goes back to sleep. I pat her on the head and whisper a thank-you. I wait for Jared to settle down, a paratrooper of love trapped behind enemy lines.

Another night I crawl into the room on my belly, a pack of diapers clenched between my teeth. I carefully lower the gate to Barak's crib, putting my T-shirt-covered thumb into the release mechanism to dampen the *Click! Wakeup-screaming!* alarms. I slide the gate down, roll Barak over, and, with practiced expertise, tear off the Velcro fastening strips with one swift motion each. I roll the diaper up and drop it by the foot of the crib—no way will I chance opening the diaper pail. Barak rolls over a few times, making it hard to apply the Balmex, and at one point, with the yellow blanket tangled up in his legs and his hips swiveling in the opposite direction of his head, I pick him up in the air, untangle him, and put him down again—a clean reboot. Rocky is finished and I admire him in the moonlight, his knees tucked into his chest, his thumb draped at the end of his pursed-open mouth, his lips twittering with sweet, congested breaths.

I worry about Barak. I worry that I favor Jared because of his squeaky-wheel approach to babyhood. I see the confident spark in Jared's eye and know he will have a very successful career as a child. He will enjoy the love of parents and family, the affection of strangers, the esteem of his peers.

Hannah, too, because of her iron will, will also enjoy a successful childhood career. Her murderous screams when food is delayed, her easy manipulation of her mother, and her natively feminine wiles serve her well.

But Barak trails the other two. He talked last and complains the least. Roni and I joke that Barak has middle-child syndrome. Safety valve and middle-child syndrome are not the harbingers of a successful baby career. Barak needs a game plan, a strategy, to help him to maximize his infancy. Toddlerhood is coming soon and I want him to be prepared.

Having failed to Ferberize Jared, there is not much I can say about my nightly missions behind baby lines. If I let Jared cry, he wakes Hannah, who has begun to copy Jared—as Roni predicted—because she sees me remove him and reacts with jealousy.

Sometimes, in the morning, I hear Jared standing silently in his crib. I peek in the room and see Jared clap his chubby little hands together. When he hears me or sees me—or, as Roni hypothesizes, smells me—he makes a squalling happy noise, and despite the fact that I am worn out, the joy on Jared's face makes me forget I am being manipulated like a marionette. Sometimes he claps his hands together when he sees me and loses his grip on the crib, falling backward and knocking himself silly. I peer down in the crib and find him laughing at his own klutziness.

"Dada!" Jared says.

Jared doesn't always want to go back to sleep. He likes to hang out and play, and after thirty minutes it is not cute anymore, especially at 2:00 A.M. Sometimes I sit him in my lap and turn on the little TV in the kitchen and try to hypnotize him. When I try to put Jared back in his crib he sometimes screams and bucks and flails around violently, like a crocodile caught in a noose.

Roni calls Jared's violent thrashings "sleep demons." If she is dozing off in bed, she will sometimes take Jared and cuddle with him. We set up a playpen as a temporary bed in the fourth bedroom. This is the "isolation booth" for a child who refuses to go back to sleep. The triplets sense my guilt over this arrangement—normal in any other home—and react with pure, distilled rage if sentenced here. The ungodly screams are too much for Roni and me to tolerate, and after a month or so, the isolation booth is abandoned, so any baby who refuses to stop screaming is rewarded with a night snuggling in the big bed between Mommy and Daddy.

The babies are eleven months old now and explode across the house. Even though they are not walking yet, they spread out far and wide to wreak havoc. We have baby-proofed the house, but you can't invasion-proof a house.

One baby can only get so far toward the front door, but three babies going in three different directions are the practical expression of chaos theory. They enjoy crawling into the pantry and knocking cans of food over like bowling pins. From the bathroom they drag out the jumbo rolls of paper towels and punch holes in the plastic and logroll themselves around. The swinging door to the kitchen is wedged open with a doorstop, but one baby working methodically can hammer out the doorstop and release the door. A small cupboard under a built-in bookcase houses games and shoes that can be scattered like grains of sand.

They pull themselves up on the living room couch and stare out the front windows onto Kraft Avenue. There are dogs and cars and children outside and usually some work papers of Mommy and Daddy that can be sent airborne or torn into interesting shapes.

Asher finally assumes his rightful station as Lord of the Babies. The babies follow him everywhere. He can address them under the flimsiest of pretexts to march them around the house in loose—i.e., crawling furiously—but dedicated formation.

"Why are the babies under the dining room table?" I ask, when I see little sneaky faces peering out from beneath the chairs.

"They're in a shark cave, and they're not allowed out, because the lead shark is hungry," Asher explains.

Of course, being Lord of the Babies has unintended consequences, such as the babies following Asher into his room uninvited. Asher's room has six-foot-high Metro shelving filled with toys, doodads, books, stuffed animals, and art supplies. The babies pile in behind him, their eyes wide with wonder, as if stumbling upon the gold vaults of El Dorado. They attempt to scale Asher's twin bed, that magical resting place of their master and lord. Jared easily pulls himself up using Asher's covers, followed by Hannah, which leaves poor Barak panting helplessly on the floor. He is either not coordinated enough or, I suspect, not motivated enough to make the climb.

"Daddy!" Asher screams. "The babies are destroying my bed!"

I explain that the babies are simply copying him and are not trying to cause any real damage. But the manic glee with which the babies invade his bed and scale his shelves contradicts their lack of ill intent.

Jared idolizes Asher. Sometimes I watch Jared when Asher is lathering the babies up with one of his drawn-out soliloquies, and the love on Jared's face is a dazzling light that illuminates everyone. When Asher gets mad and yells at Jared, Jared breaks down and sobs uncontrollably.

"Asha yet me!" Jared says, sobbing into my shoulder. He peers up from my snot-stained shirt to catch a glimpse of his tormentor and king.

As Jared follows Asher, Hannah follows Jared. If Jared wakes up early, Hannah wakes up early. If Jared is eating an apple, then an apple Hannah will have. If Jared has to move his bowels then—what a coincidence—make way for Hannah. On the odd morning when Jared sleeps late, Hannah sleeps late, too.

Asher is aware that Roni is concerned for Hannah's independence, since she is one girl among three boys, and that Jared extorts more attention from me and demands the most uppies. I begin to comprehend that the matrix of interlocking relationships is more complex than I ever anticipated. Each of the triplets will have a unique relationship with each of the others. Asher will have a unique relationship with each of the babies, as will Roni and I. The triplets, as a triangle, will have their own constantly evolving internal group dynamic. And the four kids together will array themselves against the authority of their parents. The strings of two dozen distinct relationships will intertwine in one densely emotional Jacob's ladder.

The one-year birthday mark approaches and Roni and I confront a tough decision. We are paying Rosetta and Agnes good salaries and have killed off all of our savings, not to mention missing our IRS estimated tax payments because we are out of cash. With Asher in school all day now, we only need one baby-sitter, but both of them are wonderful. We can't afford both and can't easily fire one.

Roni's friend Marcy is about to give birth to twins, and without any prompting, Rosetta volunteers to work for Marcy. Rosetta and Marcy both live in the city, they are both the quiet and considerate type, they already like each other—it works out perfectly. Agnes is wonderful with the babies and her daughter, Ronicia, is the big sister to all our kids.

The first birthday party is scheduled for a Sunday in early February. Planning for the party makes us slightly melancholy, because we realize how little we have socialized in the past year. At least Roni hangs out with her girlfriends. But my guy friends are either single and living in Los Angeles or married with kids in New Jersey. To negotiate Daddy play-date clearance is like negotiating with a mob-run labor union. I call my college buddy Dave Epstein, who has two boys and lives in central New Jersey and never calls me anymore, and ask if we will ever hang out and act stupid again.

"I don't think so," Dave says. "Let me put Charlene on the phone." Dave used to fight three or four guys at a time in tough Irish bars in Newark for fun, and now he is handing the phone to his wife.

"You can go out with your buddies anytime," Roni says. I do not accept as coincidence the bizarre emergencies that cause a cancellation whenever I organize a boys' night out.

The babies' actual birthday is the Thursday before their party, and all week long Roni crazily prepares to bake three separate birthday cakes. Two years ago she made a train cake for Asher's first birthday—three cars built from three different flavors of cake, each car decorated with different colors and flavors of cream cheese frosting, and each detailed with unique candy and other decorative items—and she internalized this accomplishment as one of her motherhood-defining rituals. She created a new homemade cake for Asher's every birthday and now she will make three.

"You don't have to make the three cakes from scratch," I say. "At least buy the cakes and then design and decorate them."

Roni won't listen. She is making three separate car cakes from scratch. My worry is that in the cake obsession the housecleaning will be forgotten until a panicky all-night cleaning marathon erupts late Saturday night. I try to forestall this by strategically cleaning the dining room and living room on Wednesday afternoon.

"I want to rearrange the living room and dining room," Roni says Wednesday night. Oh, God, I think—now she has evil powers, too.

We argue about birthday presents. Roni wants all presents held until Sunday, the day of the party. One of Roni's quirks is her habitual belatedness in giving birthday presents. She gave me my thirty-sixth birthday present well after I turned thirty-seven.

Roni says the kids will get dozens of presents and they can wait. She refuses to let them turn into gift addicts like other kids. "They're only one," I say. "We're not going to spoil them. I want them to understand that the day of their birth is an important day."

"It can be important without candy and gifts," Roni says.

"That's one of those things that's true but not true," I say.

To compromise, I am allowed to give one or two small toys and cupcakes for their actuarial birthday as long as they receive no treats Friday and Saturday. I sign off on this stipulation because, between my mom and Roni's, no shortage of treats will be suffered.

Roni and I are slightly disappointed that none of the triplets will walk by their first birthday. Barak will not even admit that walking is an activity that interests him. Hannah enjoys hanging on to the couch and standing up so she can fall back on her rear end with a satisfying thud. Jared climbs over obstacles and up and down the stairs like a jungle cat, but has not taken a single vertically integrated step.

The morning of their first birthday, I test the video camera as the kids are getting dressed with Agnes and Rosetta. Asher clowns for the camera and drags Barak and Hannah into a loud, improvised skit. Rosetta and Agnes pull Jared to his feet. Jared smiles at me with that self-knowing smile and takes one wobbly step, then another.

"Oh my God, Mommy, Jared is walking," Asher screams, and runs down the stairs, although Roni is already on the train, another milestone passing her by. Smiling right into the camera, Jared takes an incredible thirteen steps before tumbling back down to the carpet. Jared laser-beams a smile that says he understands his achievement.

Asher gives Jared high fives, and I realize he is excited because once the babies walk they will be his own personal army, available to serve him, follow him, run interference, and take the fall. These aren't just brothers and sisters anymore—they are reinforcements.

TWELVE

The Special Box

The crime scene is in a notoriously dangerous part of town. The victim lies facedown in a pool of Magic Marker ink. The three perps hide in a nearby closet, where they wrongly assume powers of invisibility, as evidenced by the giggling and whispering and sticking out of heads. The victim's family stands off to one side, tears running down his tightly drawn face.

"The marker will wash off," I explain, holding up the heavy plastic Tommy Pickles doll, maimed in five or six Crayola colors.

"That's not *the point!*" Asher says.

The babies are sixteen months old now. Asher, four, probes our system of rules and moral definitions with the vigilance of a first-year law student. Here is a clear case of criminal intent and he demands to know the repercussions. A group time-out strikes him as too lenient a sentence.

"They're going to play in time-out, so how is that punishment?" Asher says.

The triplets aggressively explore the house now and rack up a list of infractions on Asher's police blotter that grows by the day. They regard Asher's room as a utopia of toys and privilege and scale his shelves with impunity, plunder swelling their hearts. I try to explain to Asher that he is a superstar in their eyes and in their fascination they go too far, although I doubt Tom Cruise's greatest fans would throw his knickknacks down the stairs and jump up and down on his bed, screaming and thrashing.

While Asher enjoys the privacy of his own room, he prefers to hang out in the triplet's room. His personality is to seek out wherever the action is. No matter how much coercion I apply, Asher will play games or launch projects in his room only when the babies are sleeping or out of the house.

I scrub the marker off the Tommy doll's hard plastic face under Asher's watchful gaze and worry how he is handling such a monstrous adjustment—the move from city to suburbs, the start of nursery school, the loss of his old city friends, the imposition of three siblings who divide and absorb the parental attention previously lavished upon him, the new sticky-handed reign of terror.

Forget about a glass of water at night or help with a lost toy—how will Asher communicate his more subtle needs, his sadness or worry or feelings of exclusion, over the strain of our daily decibel level? Is he keeping his feelings to himself? Sometimes I look at Asher and my stomach somersaults over the stress he surely feels.

Yet Asher rarely complains about being ignored. He does well in his pre-K class academically and socially. He is verbally precocious, reads a year or two ahead of his age group, speaks a mile a minute, and is kind and considerate to the triplets 90 percent of the time. Like most four-year-olds, he a joy to be around.

Roni says Asher is lucky to have two brothers and a sister so close in age. The biggest complaint most kids have is that they are bored or want a playmate. Such words have never been uttered in our house. Our kids don't need play dates—they *are* a play date. From 7:00 A.M. to 9:30 or 10:00 P.M. something is always happening at our house, often two or three activities simultaneously. We have to tell the four kids to stop playing to get dressed, eat, drink, and go to the bathroom.

Roni points out how some of Asher's school friends—especially the only children—look back over their shoulders at our house with regret when they leave a play date. Once in a while, a kid will grab on to the porch railing when his mom shows up and scream that he doesn't want to leave. Our house is a never-ending party.

Asher and Jared's closeness includes a growing competitiveness. Jared looks the most like Asher, is the most physically skilled and the most naturally charming, making him the most immediate threat to Asher's sovereignty.

One day Asher finds Jared removing a small toy from an old party bag stashed high on his shelves. It is only a cheap plastic whistle that we forbid Asher to use inside the house. In fact, Asher never used the whistle, but this violation of his privacy drives him to distraction.

"The babies won't leave my stuff alone!" Asher complains. "It's not fair!"

I look around Asher's room, realize he has no safe harbor for his favorite belongings, and promise to find a solution for him.

Later that night the triplets are in their cribs, raking the bars and singing and screaming, heaving toys out, showing off, jumping up and down—the typical demented musical prison riot of bedtime. Asher eggs them on, a maestro of the maelstrom.

In Roni's bedroom closest I find one of those inexpensive cardboard boxes sold in camera stores for collecting photographs. Once the babies settle down I bring it in to Asher's room and we sit on the floor together.

"This will be your special box," I say. "You can put all your important stuff in here. I'm going to write your name on it." In indelible black marker I write Asher's name across the front.

"Now, you put all the stuff in here you don't want anyone else to touch, even me and Mommy, okay? It will be only for you. And we'll find a special secret place for it."

Asher holds the box in his hands, analyzing the logic of it, my little Oliver Wendell Holmes. "But the babies will open it," Asher says. "There's no lock. See?" Asher whips open the lid of the box and heaves it across the room in a deft imitation of a frenzied toddler.

I explain that the special box will be stored out of the triplets' reach. We will institute a unique off-limits policy for the special box, along with harsh penalties for special-box violations. This is tantamount to putting a flashing red sign on the box that says Open Me! but I will tackle this problem later.

Asher's imagination has been captured. I leave him to put on his PJs and brush his teeth while I call Roni for the latest law firm soap opera news. When I see that it is almost 10:00 P.M. I hang up on Roni and run into Asher's room, expecting to find him asleep on the floor, carpet fibers in his hair, a handful of toys clenched in his fists.

The tableaux spread across the floor of Asher's room is stupefying. My son has meticulously taken down the toys and knickknacks piled and strewn over the eighteen square feet of metal shelving and triaged it down to a nucleus of his most prized possessions.

Tubs of miscellaneous toys and lost toy parts have been carefully searched and resorted, piles of toys we have given up hope of restoring yet cannot bear to throw out have been stripped apart, analyzed, and catalogued with cold, clinical precision.

The crown jewels of his kingdom, the toys he is carefully layering into his special box, do not correlate to any objective commercial value or obvious emotional attachment. I see useless plastic toys taken from long-forgotten party bags and cereal boxes, an odd chess piece from a decimated chess set, a glow-in-the-dark pen that neither glows nor writes, some small, unidentifiable metal spare parts which I hope do not belong to one of Roni's toolboxes.

I quiz Asher about his methodology, gently trying to impart the safety-deposit box logic that is dictated, but Asher knows his own mind and is not easily swayed.

"I know what I want in my special box, Daddy," Asher says. "Can I just get my work done—please?"

"We have to start cleaning up," I say. It's after 10:00 P.M. on a school night.

"I need to finish this!" Asher says.

I initiated this project—and Asher is compulsive about his work—so I give in. Forty minutes later, Asher is in bed with his special box, nearly three-quarters full, balanced on his stomach. His eyes are puffy from exhaustion, but he cannot go to sleep.

"I can keep it next to me, on my pillow," Asher says.

We quietly discuss the installation of the special box. I offer to secure it high up in his closet, or on the very top shelf of his toy shelving, or in our bedroom in some unreachable place.

While aware of the threat level posed by the babies, Asher does not want his special box hidden far from view. He is worried some unnamed fate will befall it once it leaves his field of vision, a fear I understand intimately, because I routinely imagine disasters consuming my nostalgic trinkets.

Asher wants to keep the special box on his radiator cover, an idea I resist. The radiator is at triplet-reach level and the special box will sit unprotected and alone, begging to be pillaged. In the winter the contents of the special box will be cooked like salmon in tin foil. Asher is tired and irrational and insists the radiator cover is the perfect place to settle the special box, whether I approve or understand, or not.

And so begins another case of the four-year-old boy proving wiser than his father. When Asher places the special box on the radiator the next day the babies do not notice it. When they saunter into his room, Jared climbs into Asher's bed, Barak rummages through the shelves and Hannah hunts down any possible traces of candy. The special box is a giant, electric-pink elephant vibrating at a frequency only I can see.

I turn to Asher to accept his hard-earned scorn but he is too busy bossing the triplets around to savor his intellectual victory. "Let's march!" Asher insists, handing out musical instruments. The triplets follow Asher around in a dissonant frenzy of clanging and banging and hooting and broken-string twanging. When is it, I wonder, that children are corrupted by the need to say they told us so?

As the weeks go by, I remain puzzled by the triplets' indifference to the special box. How can they miss it? Is the simplest answer that Asher has hidden the box in plain sight? Or is the box somehow visually numbing? Possibly Asher has been transmitting reality-bending thought waves, like an Indian fakir.

Asher ignores the special box for days or weeks, then suddenly attacks it with a fury of activity, some invisible trick of memory sending him to action. He rarely rummages through the special box when bored, but opens and closes it to deposit new treasures. Every few months or so he spends a few hours angrily rearranging the contents, a troubling DNA refraction of Roni's folding disorder.

One day I buy Asher some Rugrats stickers for a father-son art project, but Asher insists on depositing the Rugrats stickers in his special box, where they will remain pristine and untouched.

"But I thought we'd make a card for your teacher," I say.

"No, I want to save the stickers," Asher says. He carefully puts the stickers in the special box, closes it up, and returns to the triplets' room. I stare at the special box in the empty room and wonder if I have done more harm than good.

Soon I realize that one of the duties of the special box is to be a vault for items that demand preservation. But unlike property deeds or family jewelry, whose value remains timeless over generations, many items in the special box will become dated within six months or a year. An expiration date on a child's emotional attachment to any given object passes with brutal speed.

Special-box objects expire for all kinds of reasons. Tootsie Rolls and Blow Pops and other nonhermetically sealed treats must be secretly trashed. Lion and tiger picture cards from an environmental matching game are orphaned when the remainder of the game is tossed away. One day, when he moves on to another favorite TV show, the Rugrats stickers will become as obsolete as stale candy. The special box is a finite space. Will he let me discharge expired special objects to make way for the new? Or will he cling to these special things even as they evolve into meaningless, calcified relics of old moments of whimsy?

I take intense pleasure in seeing Asher open his special box, fuss with the contents and add new treasures. In the special box I have found a concrete physical expression of my concern for his privacy and self-identity. Here is a way for him to seize back a degree of control over his life. Just as I am glad to see him spending quiet minutes in his room alone with a book or a tape, to see him quietly tend to his special box gives me great comfort.

The special box's importance becomes clear the day it disappears. One morning before school Asher wants to deposit a new toy, but I notice the special box is not on the radiator or anywhere else in his room.

Between eating breakfast, Roni leaving for work in the dust cloud of her daily list of instructions, coordinating the day's agenda with Agnes, and prepping Asher for his ride to school, I distract Asher from the situation.

I rush into the city to work and call home to ask Agnes to search for the special box in the few places my intuition says it may turn up. She has no luck. I spend the rest of the day worrying about the box and how I will explain its disappearance.

Like most kids, Asher can obsess over a problem, no matter how small, no matter how disproportionate to reality, no matter how easily solved. My day is ruined.

Where could the special box be?

"Don't worry. It will turn up," Roni says. How neatly we switch roles when the anxiety rests on the other person's shoulders.

I play out and discard all the scenarios in which the special box is accidentally and catastrophically destroyed. Roni lectures me about how things should never be moved out of their designated places. She is a firm believer in the everything-in-its-place theory of life, save for her lost car keys, money, wallet, work papers, credit cards, medical insurance card, building security card, and deathly-important phone numbers scribbled on scraps of paper, a small sample of her personal exemptions from this theory.

All day long at work my head buzzes with worry. Whenever the phone rings with a publicist trying to pitch the latest underwater camera rig or 3-D animated talking porcupine, I feel as if my head were going to explode.

"Don't you people realize the special box is missing!" I scream silently, mm-hmming and yuh-uhh-uhing my way through another conversation about the relative virtues of D-1 versus D-3 digital tape in a day of tedium that drip-drops, drip-drops, across my consciousness.

My trip home consists of two subways to Grand Central and then the Metro North train to the suburbs. Inexplicable delays block every step of the journey, as if I am in a childhood dream in which I run from a faceless, slashing killer and my feet will not work.

I must rescue that stupid box from its fate. But every malevolent force in the universe has turned out to delay, subvert, and thwart my mission. The number 2 subway express train is slower than the number 3 local. The shuttle subway train across town is having a door problem. The Metro North schedules have changed again and the Metro North train waits at 125th Street without explanation. Finally I elbow my way past a heavyset woman carrying a Zaro's shopping bag full of cakes and cookies when the train stops in Bronxville and hoof it home double-time.

The house is thoroughly untainted by special boxes. I rip sheets off beds, push dressers away from walls, circle and recircle the obvious places, as though the box will return in a flash of light from its temporary journey into an alternate universe.

After about forty-five minutes, when I am leaving to pick Asher up at an after-school play date, I suddenly see the special box in the dining room, sitting nonchalantly atop the highboy converted to arts-and-crafts storage. I don't remember putting the special box up there. I can't blame Roni or Agnes, because I am the only one who uses the space on top of the highboy. Somehow, over the last forty-eight hours, I became lost on the interstate of my mind and ditched the special box by the side of the road.

Asher does not even ask about the special box when I pick him up from school. He doesn't ask about it on the way home, during dinner, or as we put the triplets to bed.

We are playing in his room when I finally blurt out my joyous rediscovery.

"I found the special box! I can't believe you forgot about it!" I say.

Asher's face brightens as he turns to look at the box, sitting serene and undisturbed atop the radiator, where it is supposed to be. Then he goes back to the Connect Four game we are playing and cannot be bothered to think about it anymore. I am left to stew in my private humiliation over the extravagant amount of mental energy I expended, but at least the special box is back home where it belongs, safe and sound, and all seems right with the world.

Nicky pulls me into his office. He wants me on the road for two weeks in northern California, two in Los Angeles, one in the Midwest, one in the South/Southwest, and a week's worth of day trips on the East Coast. We have two major weeklong trade shows, plus three brand-new trade shows—that's a minimum of ten to eleven weeks of travel for the year. "Playtime's over," Nicky says. "You need to start making something happen." Ad pages for all the magazines in our industry sector are down again. When ad pages are down, editorial gets blamed, even in a broad recession.

I told Nicky I would spend seven to eight weeks on the road. A week a month not only turns our home upside down but delays production of the magazine. And the tone of my job has changed. More of my meetings with hardware and software companies end with my being excused to the waiting room while our ad sales rep unfolds an advertising schedule. In magazines, the attention of the editor is always the bait, but I am tired of being a giant, fat, dangling carrot. My marginal status as an industry expert— I predicted, in print, the success of *The Simpsons, Toy Story* and *Titanic* months before their first reviews—means little to my company, so how much is it supposed to mean to me?

Age: 38
Job Description: Carrot
Objective: To become a mixed green salad

On the train ride home I watch the men leaving the train in Bronxville. They wear expensive, perfectly tailored suits with French cuffs—I don't even know what a French cuff is—and wing-tip shoes by shoemakers of whom I never heard. They look perfectly content in their roles as industry titan dads. No lines of doubt crease their thin, tanned faces. Most of my male friends are lawyers or doctors or investment bankers or executives. I keep worrying that I climbed aboard the wrong train. The writer thing is juvenile. I should be wearing a suit and pulling down $100K. I am a defective money-making machine.

Since college, I have filled two dozen moving boxes with short stories, aborted novels, movie scripts, TV scripts, humor books, articles, comedy sketches, and stand-up comedy routines. I keep these boxes lined up on shelves in the basement, the pages yellowing, turning brittle and sticking together with age. I won't let Roni or the moving men even touch them—I move all of them myself, gingerly, in a rented car or step van. Each box represents hundreds or thousands of hours of work irretrievably sacrificed to no apparent end. The labels on the boxes—Scrnply, Shrt

Stry, Outlns, Ideas, Humr Bk., Random Nts.—have peeled off and died on sludge-covered concrete floors. I should have been a shrink, because the summers in Cape Cod would be perfect for us.

Roni and I were married in November 1991. We brain-stormed how to jump-start my TV and movie writing career, so I packed up and moved to Los Angeles in March of 1992. Film Tech opened an office for me and Greg Solman, my buddy (and best man at my wedding) and also our West Coast editor, on Melrose Avenue. The magazine needed more bodies on the ground in L.A, so the move worked for everyone. Alison Johns, the editor of the magazine and an old friend from college, knew I was writing scripts and winked at it, because that's how good writers stayed happy. I commuted between L.A. and New York for two years, until Roni was seven months pregnant with Asher.

During one of my trips back East I stopped in to see my mom, who lived in Langhorne, Pennsylvania, about fifteen miles south of Trenton, New Jersey. My mom had one small closet to hold all of her life's junk, most of which she jettisoned when she divorced my dad in 1978, closed up and sold our suburban house, and moved into her first apartment since she was a single girl.

During this visit I was fishing around in her closet and discovered my trash bag full of old baseball cards. This was the tip of the iceberg of my monstrous collection of base-ball, hockey, basketball, and football cards, which I began collecting in 1968 and continued through 1972. In the intervening thirty years, this bag had been reduced by a flood and other unfortunate events.

My sports card collection was childish in nature but not in scope. As a kid, I had five or six large boxes—equivalent to the box a nineteen-inch television set is packed in—filled with sports cards, some 150,000 or so cards. I spent all my allowance and birthday money on sports cards. I bought so many cards that I sold the single sticks of pink bubble gum from the wax packs at school to make money to buy even more cards. I had whole sets of Topps baseball, football, basketball and hockey from 1969 to 1971. I remember stacks of the beautiful pink-backed 1969 cards with Mickey Mantle and Roberto Clemente and Willie Mays. I even sent away in the mail to buy older cards, from the turn-of-the-century cigarette cards to classic cards from the 1950s. Old friends vividly remember my card collection. My buddy Mike Posner, now a lawyer in Miami, clearly recalls how I wanted to borrow $100,000 to buy the famous Honus Wagner cigarette card in 1971.

I looked through the water-stained cards spread over my mom's coffee table. There were four 1968 Nolan Ryan rookie cards, purple with water stains. A 1965 Willie Mays with a rip. A large number of the black-bordered 1971 baseball cards survived, but none of my hockey, football, or basketball cards survived. I began to read up on the 1980s sports-card-collecting explosion. As a poor single guy, I did not pay attention to this kind of financially-speculative, Baby Boomer nostalgia trip.

My mom felt terrible about the cards.

"I'm sorry I didn't save them for you. I guess I wasn't thinking about it," my mom said.

I felt worse for making my mother feel guilty. She spent her whole life devoted to my brother and me and did nothing wrong. She had to collapse a four-bedroom house with a full basement down into a one-bedroom apartment in the middle of a nasty divorce, and I was away that summer and couldn't even help pack up the house. Why hadn't I taken my cards with me? I saved boxes of my old LPs and even a box of worthless 7-Eleven Slurpee cups with baseball stars on them.

I decided to blame my dad, because he actually gave away the boxes of my sports cards to the man who helped him move out of our old house. Meanwhile, he kept hundreds of boxes of his own garbage—camera parts and tools and books and broken film developers and tangled pieces of holographic equipment.

"You kept your stupid old Sears tool cabinets," I told my dad. "One box of those old baseball cards would be worth fifty or one hundred grand today!"

"I'm sorry," said my dad, gravely. "I made a lot of mistakes. I wish I could do a lot of things differently," he said. Then my dad launched into a staggeringly complex monologue about how his life hadn't worked out as he had hoped. The jobs, the stock market, his glaucoma, his asthma, his back, his allergies, the house, his job selling stereo equipment, the bills, the stock market, their divorce, his enlarged heart and his many brushes with death, the rare, lingering illnesses which doctors could not diagnose, the Byzantine plotlines of how the Philadelphia public school system crucified him . . .

"I was just kidding, Dad," I said.

"You boys have no idea what my life has been like," my dad said. "Nothing I did ever worked out. No matter how hard I tried, I always ended up going backwards. . . ."

"Don't get him started," said my brother, Paul, younger by eighteen months and a successful lawyer who lives in

Anchorage, Alaska. Paul collected sports cards with me as a kid, but never said a word about them once he left home for college. Paul never looked back, always pushing forward.

Seeing the residue of my old card collection at my mom's apartment triggered something insane inside me. After returning to Los Angeles, instead of trying to meet agents or producers, I drove around to tag sales in Encino and West Covina, hunting baseball cards. I fantasized about buying boxes of vintage baseball cards for five dollars at obscure garage sales.

This fantasy was as idiotic as wishing you could travel back in time and buy van Gogh's paintings for ten dollars. By 1992, every American was hip to the value of baseball cards. Little kids would try to sell me a crumpled-up 1974 Reggie Jackson for one hundred dollars. It was madness.

But my obsession couldn't be stopped. I lied to Roni about my whereabouts and went to sports card shows in Pasadena. Some of my friends found this behavior fascinating, and offered their own analyses, most of which centered on my attempt to recapture some lost aspect of my childhood. Some said it was an early midlife crisis. I don't know if any of this was true, but I'll say this—I wanted my goddamn fucking baseball cards back. Sometimes I opened my eyes in the morning literally mouthing the words "Baseball cards! Baseball cards! Baseball cards!"

I had vivid, recurring dreams of the house I grew up in on Thrush Lane in Huntingdon Valley, Pennsylvania, a Philadelphia suburb, from 1969 to 1978. I dreamed about my bedroom closest, where I kept my cards in giant cardboard boxes.

In my dreams, floodwaters rose through the house and roared in from the windows and poured down from the roof. I would become conscious that I was dreaming and clutch the boxes of baseball cards in my arms, praying I might be able to pull them back out to the present day and rescue them, if only I could hold on tightly enough to escape the quicksand gravity of my dream.

THIRTEEN

Lost in the Supermarket

Jared looks over his shoulder and smiles his golden boy smile. He is going to run, so I preemptively chase him.

The babies are eighteen months old now and we are outside Starbucks at the end of cookie time. Jared bolts up the main walkway, to my right, toward Park Place. Barak shouts "Let's go," and he and Hannah scamper down the steps to my left, toward Kraft Avenue. Three kids head in two different directions at the same time.

I knew this day would come. I am outnumbered.

The triplets discovered their land legs two months ago, but not the power they wield as a group. Numerical superiority counts for a lot in war and parenting. In most large families, the older kids help maintain order, but with triplets the dynamic is the opposite. Three kids the exact same age are a breakaway republic, and as they giggle and scoot away I know my control over them has moved from the physical to the psychological. I blast through the bushes and cut the three of them off at the corner. They laugh at me as I huff and puff, peat moss and dirt kicked up over my pants and shirt.

I lecture them about running into the street and we watch cars drive by. I put their hands on parked cars to show them the danger. The car is good when it takes us places, but is a screeching death machine when you are walking. A car is like—

"Daddy?" Jared says, smiling.

I know what he's thinking. "Let's go!" Barak says, and all three race up the block.

They still believe I am bigger and faster and stronger and smarter, but the more they test their freedom and physical maturity the closer they will come to the sad, baggy-panted truth. My job as parent requires me to encourage their independence, so I am writing the script for my own fall from power.

Roni frowns at the way the kids explode across the house, the playground, and the Starbucks. She wants to keep them confined but still stimulated. She wants a new mode of transportation, a vehicle to make the babies more interactive with their environment. Months of research lead her to the conclusion we need a wagon.

No ordinary wagon will do. Forget the plastic wagon, the Radio Flyer wagon, the Toys "R" Us wagon. Roni wants a true farmer's red wagon. A wagon that will cart off a dead horse and bear crops to market.

Roni discovers her dream wagon on an Internet site that distributes Amish-made merchandise. The wagon has four inflatable tires, removable barn-red side rails, and holds fifteen hundred pounds of payload. Roni outfits the wagon with Fischer-Price plastic booster seats with seat belts.

The wagon is another ungovernable monstrosity in the litany of Roni's Frankensteinian design schemes. I nearly open a hernia trying to lift it into the back of the Chevy Suburban. When I stop the wagon on the street, it smashes into the back of my legs with unstoppable momentum, gouging out my pulpy leg flesh. I mock the red wagon, even though I know Roni loves it. I crack that she loves the wagon from afar, not having to haul it around like Jethro Clampett.

"This is the dumbest thing I ever saw," I say. "We're never going to use it."

"I love it," Roni says.

"That's because you're not pulling it," I mutter.

"What?" she says.

"Nothing," I mumble, kicking at the dirt.

"Just give it a few weeks," Roni says, with her annoyingly cheery optimism. "Remember what you said about the Italian baby carriage?"

Naturally, after a few weeks, pulling the kids around town in the red wagon becomes the highlight of my day. I master the subtleties of gravity, acceleration, and local topography. The triplets ride, facing front, lined up three in a row, like passengers on a log flume. Barak sits in front, Hannah in the middle, Jared in the back. When I remove one of the side panels, Asher sits in the middle and rides side saddle.

If the blue baby carriage put us on the local news, the red wagon is *60 Minutes*. Everyone in Bronxville stops to comment how the babies have grown up and what a brilliant innovation the wagon is. One warm Saturday morning in early summer I fight Roni for the black metal handle as we walk the kids around town.

"Say you were wrong," Roni says, holding the handle behind her back, trying to blackmail a kiss out of me. If not for my humiliating gooberisms, our sex life would be nonexistent.

"You were wrong," I say.

"Daddy—that's not fair!" shouts Asher, our resident moralist. "Tell Mommy you're wrong!" Asher stands with hands on hips, demanding action.

Roni basks in the power of their unholy alliance. Now Asher switches allegiance like a free agent in baseball. Except Asher's currency is morality, and the older he gets, the more rigid his posturing.

"I was wrong," I say to Roni. I will do anything to let this moment pass. Plus, I want back control of the wagon. I want the handle. I need that handle.

Asher walks alongside the wagon, pushes from behind, or rides on the side with his feet dangling. On a flat stretch, with gravity neutralized, Asher pulls the wagon by himself. The image of my four-year-old son pulling this massive Amish load-bearing vehicle prompts passersby to stop and take snapshots of us. I stand and wait while cameras are fished out of tissue-clogged bags and glove compartments.

Senior citizens are irresistibly motivated to ask us, "Do you have room for one more in there?"

"I charge by the mile," I say. The line always gets a laugh.

The Big Red Wagon makes exploring the local supermarket a central ritual. Roni is furious when she discovers I am taking the kids to the supermarket—and in the wagon! I have complained for years about how much I hate supermarkets. This betrayal is worse than an affair with another woman, which she could forgive as a predictable failure of gender. Taking the kids to the supermarket for entertainment purposes is an inexcusable stab in the back.

"I can't believe you!" Roni says, waving a stack of crumpled, stained Food Emporium receipts. "You never take me to the supermarket!"

The absurdity of an accusation has no relationship to its marital importance. When Roni is this angry I am guilty.

I apologize for my ignorance and insensitivity and the next day I pick Roni up at the train station with the babies loaded in the red wagon. When Roni steps off the train the babies scream "Mommy" and hold out their arms. Roni squeals with excitement and I notice the sideways, envious glances of the other moms, most of them loaded down with bags from a day of shopping on Madison Avenue. It strikes me now that Roni never talks to the other moms on the train, that she feels estranged and isolated from them. I see the line of gleaming BMWs and Mercedes-Benzes and Jags with the dads or housekeepers waiting behind the wheel and the tall blond kids sitting up straight in the backseats in their horse-farm or Monet-themed PJs, and I imagine how much Roni hates getting off the train every night with the Wall Street guys in their $250 shirts.

"Who wants to go to the supermarket?"

Roni and the four kids shoot up their hands and scream "Me!"

Roni pulls the red wagon out of the parking lot, and when she turns around to smile at the kids she looks twenty years younger.

·   ·   ·

At eighteen months, the triplets territorialize every aspect of their lives. No trading of seats in the red wagon is tolerated. Even if someone is sick or sleeping, their assigned seat is sacrosanct. Simply stepping on another seat to climb into your own causes an angry fusillade of screaming and name calling.

Barak is by far the most vigilant. He is the Ayatollah of seat sanctity. If Jared or Hannah climbs into or over Barak's seat for any reason, Barak goes berserk and retaliates with a savage kicking or biting attack. Sometimes Jared will gently tease Barak, reaching out and barely touching the edge of Barak's seat, and I have to move Jared to another location for his own protection.

Fighting to defend the front seat of the red wagon coincides with an explosion in Barak's personality. Our worries about Barak playing third banana to Jared and Hannah evaporate in the flowering of his highly complex character. Barak has become a serious collector of small, worthless objects, which he protects with ferocity and passion. This is strangely similar to what Asher did when he was the same age, and the junk Asher collects now in his special box. Barak has also developed a silly streak a mile wide, and enjoys babbling nonsensical phrases—sounds, poems, gibberish, strings of broken conversation—at all hours of the day and night. He makes jokes and repeats words in a mocking, bizarre manner. He enjoys making faces at me, other kids, even total strangers.

Barak shot up in height and towers over Jared and Hannah. He has a mop of thin dirty-blond hair, the lightest complexion of the group and is sometimes mistaken for an older brother of Jared.

Barak loves animals and insects and in the warm

weather picks up ants and beetles and lets them run across his naked chest. Barak has also developed a fondness for wearing Hannah's and Roni's clothes. He enjoys putting on Roni's high heels and clomping through the house, putting on various items of Hannah's plastic jewelry, sometimes fighting for the right to wear a particularly funky piece. Barak will walk around in high heels and plastic pearls and recite nonsensical verse out of Lewis Carrol. After one of Barak's bizarre monologues, Roni and I will just stare at each other and smile with disbelief.

About twice a day, I navigate the four kids and the red wagon through the doors of the local Food Emporium.

"Bagels!" the babies shout at the baked goods that greet every shopper. They lean out of their seats and try to rip the plastic bakery bags from the dispenser.

I position the wagon away from the bagel display, yet not too close to the muffins on the opposite side. I made that mistake once and muffins flew through the air like antiaircraft fire. This is my supermarket adventure—to steer the babies through the labyrinth of retail America without creating a disaster.

Asher leads the babies in chanting for bagels. I explain that we buy our bagels fresh at the bagel store. These pathetic supermarket bagels are doomed malingerers serving out the end of their day-old life spans.

I attempt to swing past the Bakery Lady undetected, but she rushes forward to offer free cookies. The Bakery Lady is in her seventies, about four feet ten, with a deep voice and copper-colored hair, a lost descendant of the Emerald City of Oz.

Our daily ritual dovetails with the Bakery Lady's, who

greets our arrival with fanfare. She is so sweet and guileless that I feel badly about trying to sneak past her. Sometimes I plan snacks defensively around the Bakery Lady, because she will not be denied. Today the Bakery Lady offers small petit-fours with different-colored layers and a chocolate coating.

"What it is?" asks Hannah, suspicious but excited.

"I have no idea, I say. "Try it."

Asher shoves the entire cookie into his mouth. "Who wants to give me a bite of cookie for a sticker?" Asher says, trying to scam the babies out of their windfall.

Jared pushes the cookie into his pants pocket. "Saving it," Jared says. He looks very serious. He doesn't need this dessert; he will enjoy it at a more opportune moment. I do not have the heart to tell him the cookie has just been reduced to crumbs.

We swing through the fruit and produce aisle and I pick up the weirder-looking fruits and vegetables and entertain the kids. They handle a pomegranate, probably a mistake, but no one punctures it.

Jared points to a rutabaga. "What it does?" he says.

I demonstrate radicchio, endive, kale, collard greens, turnips, parsnips, and curly parsley. Asher eggs me on, a natural comic conspirator. "Put this on your head," Asher says, handing me a bunch of curly parsley. "It will look good on your bald head."

As I bag up our apples and pears and grapes, pints of strawberries suddenly make suicide leaps from the displays. Barak has corkscrewed around to sweep strawberry containers off the shelf. I catch three plastic containers before they hit the floor. Hannah comes up with a fistful of grapes.

"No!" I say. "Give me those, or no grapes."

There is silence. On a hot day, the kids devour two pounds of grapes.

"Give Daddy the grapes!" Asher says. Luckily, he also is in a grape phase, or the grapes would be crushed underneath the wheels of the wagon. The babies comply.

Jared spots a display containing cut-up cantaloupes pierced with toothpicks. "Daddy, lopes," Jared says. They love cantaloupe but I read something, somewhere, about E. coli and presliced fruit. The half-forgotten reference makes up in epidemiological severity what it lacks in factual clarity. Plus, unknown persons have touched the cantaloupe samples, which skeeves me out.

After a brief detour at the lobster tanks, and a chaotic marine-life Q&A session ("Can lobsters read?" "Are they being bad?"), we approach the red meat display case. The butcher's station features a platter of freshly cooked Italian sausage, which I dispense on toothpicks. They blow furiously on the little treats.

"It's not that hot," I say, but the blowing is integral to the tasting experience. The kids huff and puff for a few minutes and then strip off the meat.

"More, please," Asher says, stabbing me with a toothpick.

"I don't know," I say. "It's very fatty."

"It is bad?" says Jared. He eyes his barely nibbled sausage slice warily.

"Oh, Daddy, I'm so *hungry*," Asher says. "You can't just go around letting little kids *starve*, you know."

Each kid tackles one more slice of sausage as I meander down the back wall of the market, looking for safe passage. I am examining a frozen turkey when I hear laughing.

Barak has stuck his hand into the organic chicken display and is tearing at the packages. I grab his hand and immobilize it, checking the chicken packs for damage. One plastic cover is ripped open, and the top packages are slick with chicken juice.

If over-fondled fruit presents a health problem, raw chicken juice might as well be Ebola virus floating up from freshly killed monkeys. "Don't move your hand!" I say to Barak. I look around for a Food Emporium employee, a mom, a priest—anyone who might provide a wipe or paper towel.

What is the worst possible thing my son could do?

Barak tries to lick his chicken-juiced hand.

"Stop it!" I say. When I speak harshly or with impatience, Barak is the first to burst into tears, so I cringe for his reaction. Instead of crying, Barak cackles back at me. "Lickies, lickies!" he says, waggling his tongue. Barak laughs hysterically and gives me a grin of demonic pleasure, then proceeds to struggle his tongue toward his hand.

"Rocky's not behaving," Asher explains to Jared and Hannah.

I look Barak up and down. The most docile and laidback of the triplets, to his recent personality transformations he has added a wild Dennis the Menace streak.

Because Barak has been the most obedient, the most willing to wait for attention of any kind, I am reluctant to punish him. I want to encourage his bursting independence. Of course, licking raw chicken juice is not the ideal outlet for his self-expression.

While I hold Barak's hand immobilized, looking for an exit strategy, Asher begins to yell, "Lick it! Lick it!"

Jared and Hannah join in. "Lick your hand! Lick your hand!" they sing.

Barak sings "La-rah-lurll, la-lee" and takes swooping licks at his contaminated hand. Brilliantly, he licks my hand in big dog slurps in an effort to loosen my grip. I don't know whether to scream or laugh. If I let go for one second, he will slurp raw chicken juice into his mouth.

"Are these twins?" asks a woman dressed in powder blue.

Hannah has removed her safety belt and is standing on the top of the wagon rails, about to tumble over onto the floor. "Look me, Asher," she says. "I high in the sky."

I grab Hannah by the shirt. Now I am stretched out between Barak and Hannah, both hands full of misbehaving child. I have no more arms to spare.

The woman in blue is smiling and waiting for an answer.

"Triplets," I say.

"Oh, my!" the woman says. "I'll bet you and your wife stay very busy." She smiles at us, blinking big Mr. Magoo blinks.

"Everyone sit down, or no treats for two days!" I threaten.

"Daddy, we already *had* a treat," Asher reminds me.

Barak is neutralized after I send Asher down the baby aisle to find alcohol wipes. We escape the dried foods aisle after moderate damage—several bags of torn-open green lentils pour down like rain—and face the deadliest aisle of all: Breakfast cereals.

The cereal aisle is the ultimate test of parental endurance. I look for anything healthy on sale—Smart Start, Just

Right, low-fat granola. We don't go through cereal, we terrorize it. Now that Barak has also become the pickiest eater, he sometimes eats cold cereal for three straight meals and a snack. We cannot pay retail for cereal.

"I want that," Asher says, pointing to Count Chocula.

"You never even tasted it," I say.

"Daddy, want that," Jared says, pointing to a cereal that looks like chocolate chip cookies. I check the ingredients. They might as well make cereal out of pure crack cocaine. Crackies.

"Lucky Charms, Lucky Charms!" shout Hannah and Barak, pointing at Asher's favorite cereal, which they demand so often that I ration it out.

"No," I say, to all requests. Jared begins to bawl furiously.

"Want Lucky Charms!" he wails. He raises his arms up in dramatic submission. "Uppie!" he cries.

"No uppies," I say.

Hannah holds a box of Sugar Smacks. "Snacks," she says.

Asher stashes two boxes of Fruit Loops in the wagon and tries to hide them behind his legs.

"Are you kidding?" I say.

"What?" Asher says.

I ate Fruit Loops as a kid but cannot believe how disgusting they are. Is this hypocrisy or just too much information?

"No fair, no fair, no fair in your *underwear!*" Asher chants, banging on the wagon.

Hannah starts bawling. "Uppie!" she says. She worries I will pick up Jared and is launching a preemptive strike.

"No, *me* uppie," Jared calls back, looking suspiciously at

his sister. Jared and Hannah work themselves up into a froth of jealousy over the awarding of theoretical advantages. I really want to pick Jared up, because I know he is upset, but I cannot dare invoke a window rattling tantrum from Hannah.

"Daddy, just let everyone buy *one* cereal they want, and we can get *out* of here, okay?" Asher lectures.

"Who's the boss around here?" I say.

"I am," Asher says.

Staring me in the eye, Asher then points commandingly—arm extended with military precision—at the box of Lucky Charms. For greater effect, he raises his arm and lowers it back into pointing position.

I turn away and swallow a laugh. Asher is so naturally bossy and controlling, I cannot possibly contribute to this behavior. "All right. Who wants Lucky Charms?" I say.

"Hmm," Asher says, behind me.

Now I have Jared and Hannah's attention.

"Want it now!" says Barak. "Little baggie, please?"

I was going to buy Lucky Charms anyway, I tell myself.

The last aisle has dairy on one side, bread, coffee, peanut butter, and jelly on the other. It is the widest aisle, an oasis of calm. Seeing that they are temporarily out of range, the babies relax. But when I take the organic milk a short battle ensues over the custody of the two half-gallon cartons.

"Daddy," Asher says. "I have to make a poopie."

I have carefully stashed about $80 worth of groceries into the wagon, but we are closer to home than the nearest public restroom. The checkout lines are three carts deep. What am I going to do—extract everything from the wagon, dump it on the floor in one ungrateful heap, and run out the door? The return trip will consume an hour.

"Can you wait five minutes?" I ask Asher. "I promise to hurry."

What am I saying? That a painful intestinal urge can be *decreased* by sitting and waiting? What kind of fatherly oversight is that? When I need to go, it would take an F-15 Tomcat to keep me out of the bathroom.

"I don't know," Asher says. Half the time, after we rush to a public restroom and I frantically sanitize the toilet, he says the urge has passed by like a summer cloud.

Jared and Hannah balance half gallons of milk on the edges of their seats. Barak whines, over and over, "My turn, Daddy, my turn."

"Pick out some yogurt," I say to Asher, hoping to distract him.

Asher selects Trix yogurt with sugar sprinkles stashed in a special lid. We then wheel into a checkout line that has dwindled to two people, each with partially filled carts. I have a chance.

"Are you okay?" I ask Asher.

He scrunches up his face in discomfort. "Yes," he says.

"If it's an emergency, we'll run right out of here," I say.

"That's okay, Daddy. I think it went away," he says. I'm happy for the break, but I worry where, exactly, it went.

The checkout girls wave to the kids as we inch forward. To avoid the checkout gauntlet of candy and gum and toys, I normally wheel the wagon around the aisles and alongside the exit door, near the Lotto machine. But the last aisle is blocked off, so I am trapped in line with the wagon, which barely clears the sides. I deliver the standard no-grabbing lecture and the kids nod with oh-so-sincere nods. To keep them busy, I make them load our items onto the conveyor belt.

Jared and Hannah haul up the milk containers halfway, groaning to show off. Asher unloads the yogurt, Barak hands me bananas and grapes. When I fish around for my discount card I see a flash of motion out of the corner of my eye.

"No!" I say. Hannah dumps fistfuls of Bubble Yum onto the floor. Barak tears open a bag of peanut M&Ms. Jared confidently tosses packs of Dentyne gum over the display and into the next checkout line. I grab at their hands, but, as I lean over the wagon, Barak, who sits in the first seat and blocks me in the narrow space, stuffs a pack of Rollos down my shirt, then licks my nose.

I yank on the wagon handle, but with less than a half-inch clearance on each side, the wagon is jammed in tight. The babies are whooping with checkout fever.

They are drunk on their misbehavior. I make severe threats—no Rugrats, no candy, no Big Bed—but they ignore me. Barak absentmindedly kicks me in the testicles.

I stagger back a few steps. Not an engine room hit, but the ship is taking on water. I yank the wagon free and pull it clear to the Lotto machine, where the kids smack the large, blinking buttons. Walking like I have hot shrapnel in my side, I slide my debit card through the card reader.

"Cute kids!" the girl chirps. "Cash back?"

"Mmm-nn," I say, bending down to sweep up the carnage of gum and candy with starbursts popping in my eyes. The assistant manager, who I see six days a week, waves me away.

"Don't worry," he says, brooming the packs into a box. He is friendly and polite and helpful, even after I update him about the damage to his bean aisle. Sometimes I fantasize about being a powerful CEO so I can give jobs to hardworking people like this man.

"They're having some fun with you," he says, smiling.

"I guess you don't baby-sit on the side," I joke. Then I worry this might sound offensive—racially, sexually, culturally. You never know. This man has always been so helpful and calm and sweet to us, and now I say something that might hurt his feelings. Then again, maybe I haven't done anything, and all my blood has rushed to my testicles. When you spend all day with children, you forget what passes for adult conversation.

I take deep breaths. A wave of nausea breaks over me and recedes.

The assistant manager is called away and I grab my bags, but not in time to stop Barak from yanking on the wagon's metal handle, which I have idiotically left propped up in the air against the rug-cleaning-machine display.

The handle falls backward and nails Barak squarely on the forehead. I pick him up while he pitches into hysteria. "Get that man I was just talking to," I tell Asher. "Tell him I need some ice and paper towel."

"Can I get a candy bar?" Asher says.

He'll be a lawyer, like his mother, I think. "I need your help now!" I say. "Please."

Asher surveys the situation. "Oh, *all right*," he says, rolling his eyes, as though he were Ricky Ricardo, forced to bail Lucy out of yet another ridiculous predicament.

Customers stare at me with beady bird eyes. No one else is holding a screaming toddler with a red welt rising on his forehead—not in Bronxville, where we are closer to poor white trash than upper middle class.

I cradle Barak, check him for blood, tell him he is my Special Rock Man. He will have a red welt on his head. I feel him slide out of his panic and relax in my arms.

"We wants treats," Hannah reports.

Jared digs in his pocket, searching for his cookie, his face twisting with disappointment.

Up ahead, approaching the manager's station, Asher turns around and looks at me to make sure I am watching him. He hates to be left alone and is performing with unusual bravery. I smile and wave at my little helper, my throat clenching. How many times will this little man rescue me before he leaves for college?

FOURTEEN

Something in the System

"What do you think about moving to Bali?" Roni asks one hot July day as we watch the kids splash around under the Elmo sprinkler. Roni knows a family that lives half the year in Bali, then half the year in New York, selling South Pacific trinkets. She explains the premise of travel, adventure, furniture storage, home schooling, lower taxes, and tropical fruit marinades.

"I don't know," I say. "Maybe we should take some quiet time."

"You're like an old lady," Roni says. "You never want to try anything new."

The babies are nineteen months old, and our eight-year roller-coaster ride slows down for just a moment.

We spend the summer on day trips, at museums, playgrounds, and splashes under the sprinklers. The quiet is short-lived. Nicky fires me in the middle of August.

Alison, the editor before me and my close friend, was a single woman who proudly boasted she never wanted kids.

The woman Nicky hires to replace me is married but cannot have children. Both women are tall, thin, and attractive, catnip to the computer geeks who buy advertising space. Both worked hard, were loyal, and suffered no family distractions—just like men. Instead of a glass ceiling, I hit the Huggies ceiling. When I made my kids a priority, my days were numbered. Despite the New Age management rhetoric in magazines like Fast Company, men cannot really juggle life and home issues, because if home life interferes, you are out, like old toast.

Nicky handles my firing with predictable oafishness. At 11:00 A.M. he tells me to be out by 1:00 P.M. I pack up eleven years' worth of junk into two garbage bags, abandoning dozens of personal items—toys, movie posters, bottles of wine, publicity photos, magazine clips, paperweights, a decade of funky mementos. I am not angry, just frustrated that I did not quit on my own terms and tell Nicky what I thought about him. You can't tell someone what you really think about them when you're frantically trying to delete eleven years of letters, work, and e-mail from your hard drive and remember where your *Simpsons* animation cel was stashed. Once the shock wears off, I feel relieved.

On the train ride home I worry Roni will freak out, but her reaction is uncharacteristically Zen-like. She says things happen for a reason, that I have been given a chance to change course, and demands that I finish my horror screenplay. For all our fights, and all the ways we fail to appreciate one another, I feel now, as if for the first time, the depth of Roni's support for my career as a writer. I wonder if she feels sorry she married a struggling writer and not a doctor or lawyer or real estate developer. She let me be myself all these years. Now the lawyers in her office joke that she is supporting her unemployed husband. We pay a price for going our own way, but it is the only way we know how to go.

My mother worries. She always worked and knows how rough unemployment can be. I reassure her that I am happy to pursue long-delayed writing projects.

"I'm still going to worry," she says.

"You're good at what you do," I say.

I finish my horror screenplay, *Hee-Hee's Coming*, the story of a powerful evil force that threatens a young single dad and his little boy. The idea came from Asher. One day, when Asher was eighteen months old, he claimed a friend told him that "Hee-Hee" was going to get him. I loved the creepiness of the name Hee-Hee and the story flowed naturally.

Roni finds two women producers in L.A. who want to option the script. The bad news is they are only going to pay twenty dollars. Not exactly the front-page *Variety* fantasy, but "the girls" love the story and plan an aggressive sales campaign.

Asher begins his second year of pre-K in Scarsdale at the innovative and caring private school where the annual tuition is triple what I paid for a year at Rutgers.

In October, my mom calls to say that her latest EKG shows evidence of two undiagnosed heart attacks. She has been unusually tired over the past year, and I have nagged her to change her blood pressure medication and find a new cardiologist. Now her cardio team wants to do an angiogram.

In early November I go to Philly to escort my mom to her angiogram. She is sixty-seven, barely five feet tall, with dark hair and a crinkly lifetime tan. Her mother, my grandmother Bessie, is ninety-five and still going strong. Longevity is on our side.

My mother's internist is snotty and aloof. Her cardiology team offers conflicting answers about her history. I quickly become frustrated with the whole situation. The angiogram shows severe blockages in three arteries. My mom needs a triple bypass.

Back at my mother's apartment, I grocery shop and cook a dinner of sautéd chicken with peppers and onions. We watch TV and talk about life. She shows me some family jewelry she wants me to have, but I accuse her of being morbid.

"If you think you're getting out of free baby-sitting now that you're retired, you're kidding yourself," I say.

I sleep on the fold-out couch where I have crashed for years. I always pushed her to move to a more upscale apartment, but it has a shabby, lived-in quality that makes it warm and welcoming, a home for me no matter my age or marital status. We were always very close—I was a classic mama's boy, until I was old enough to hit keg parties— but since I moved to New York in 1982 I come home less and less frequently.

Back in New York, the NYU Hospital cardiac surgeon impresses me with his thorough questioning of my mother's medical history. But the surgery makes me nervous. My mom is a lifelong smoker and I worry her anxieties will complicate her post-op recovery. The cardiac surgeon's questions reveal that my mom is taking sleeping pills and antidepressants, a total surprise to me. She kept the bad news under wraps—her lifelong MO—so as not to make me concerned.

My mother lived in generic one-bedroom apartments since 1978, worked in tedious, unrewarding jobs, struggled to make new friends. She never got the life she deserved. I wanted her to travel and pursue long-denied interests. To know she is fighting depression instead of line dancing and taking scuba-diving lessons—whatever she wants—is intensely upsetting. I scan the last twenty years for signs I missed. . . .

But we will have time to discuss her life plans during cardio rehab. I need to stay positive. The survival rate for this cardiac surgeon is 98 percent. My mom just retired from a job at GMAC finance after working like a dog for forty-five years. She has five amazing grandchildren to enjoy. These are the golden years for which she toiled so diligently. How could God let anything happen to her now?

We are expecting twenty-five people for Thanksgiving. One night Roni sucks me into a fight over some trivial serving platter decision and I yell that this could be my mother's last Thanksgiving. Roni says I am being melodramatic and my mom will be fine.

Roni nitpicks, I worry. When Barak has a fever I worry about encephalitis or some rare emerging tropical virus and stay up all night feeling his forehead. I worry about mosquitoes and ticks and rabid bats and radon and killer mold and mad cow disease and terrorism and bad potato salad and estrogen in the Tupperware and freak playground accidents and seat belts failing and solar radiation and dying suddenly in my sleep. I worry that my anxiety lives deep in my genes and I am passing it down, but even if it is purely behavioral I am still dumping it on them, like saggy old luggage, a lose-lose scenario that begs the question of whether or not we enjoy free will.

My mom doesn't want to travel now that her surgery has been scheduled. She will eat turkey with my grandmother Bessie, and warns me not to worry.

"That's like Michael Jackson telling someone not to have plastic surgery," I say.

"Well, I don't want you worrying about me," she says.

"I'm worrying," I say. "It's payback."

"Worry about Asher and the babies," my mom says.

My brother, Paul, flies in from Anchorage and we check my mother into NYU Hospital. The three of us tease each other and enjoy an impromptu family reunion. "For an extra five thousand dollars, they'll make you two inches taller," I tell her. "When you wake up, you'll be able to speak Japanese," Paul says. We arm wrestle on her hospital bed and ask the interns smart-ass questions—How much do you weigh? What floor do the famous people stay on? It amazes me how different we are and how much fun we have together, at least until my mom or I unintentionally break one of Paul's rules or interfere with his workout schedule, and then his garrulous, can-do nature slams shut like a warehouse door. I bring lunch in for my mom, but the pasta salad is too spicy. I feel horrible—this is her last regular meal before surgery Tuesday morning.

On Thursday morning—two days late, after my mom is bumped from the OR four times—she finally has the bypass. After eleven hours Paul and I get the call—"textbook surgery," the cardiac surgeon says. We can see her in a few hours. Paul and I hug like two little boys. My logic is vindicated—this is not my mother's time to go. It didn't help that the hospital made numerous mistakes—such as scheduling my mom for a valve replacement (which she was not getting) or sending a doctor in to give her post-surgery breathing therapy the night she checked in—which made Paul and me briefly debate changing hospitals.

I see her in cardiac recovery, flat on a gurney, out cold, the breathing tube jammed down her throat, and cry like a little boy. I am so grateful to see her alive, and when they took her down for surgery the last thing she said was that she would always be there to watch over Paul and me, and she looks so close to death—immobile, pale, covered by a white sheet. I sit with her and hold her hand for hours as she wakes from the surgery. Paul and I take turns staying with her.

I carry alcohol-based disinfectant gel and scrub my skin raw when I see my mom, afraid I will transfer a cold or virus from the red-hot epidemiological volcano that is our house.

My mother does not want to touch me, either. She worries I will carry a hospital-borne infection home to the kids. So now I kiss her on the cheek and on the leg and the top of her head and hold her by the elbow, hovering like a moth on a lightbulb. "I could hang over your bed from a rope," I say. My mom laughs. She always was an easy audience. This is the essence of my mother, to always worry about someone else before herself.

In the ICU we catch up on family gossip. I describe Roni's obsession with refolding towels and how she talks to herself in the kitchen and survives for days on cream cheese and crackers. We make fun of the ICU nurses, especially the nurse who eats salsa and chips despite the prominent *No Food or Drink!* signs.

I miss hanging out with my mom. To Roni, I am a work in progress, and to the kids, I am a glorified slave. My mom is the only person in the world afflicted with the opinion that I am perfect. I might not deserve the spotlight, but the light sure is warm.

My mother was five feet even and ninety-five pounds when I was born, a C-section at nine pounds, ten ounces. "You were the biggest baby in the nursery," she says, a story she never tires of repeating. "The other mothers would point at you and say, 'What's that six-month-old baby doing in the nursery?' "

Asher was a C-section at nine pounds, four ounces, had thick black hair and also looked like the oldest baby in the nursery. Asher looked exactly like me—our baby pictures are identical—and my mother's first grandchild was the apple of her eye. I joked she was having estrogen flashbacks. We teased her and called Asher "Little Bruce" whenever she held him.

My mom was ferociously protective of Asher. If we took Asher out in the stroller during a nap, she became incensed. "I would *never* take you boys out when you were sleeping!" she said. I was dumbstruck. My mother hadn't criticized me since . . . well, ever. I was proud to feel her maternal wrath.

My mom's blanket of worry folded neatly over me to include Asher. When we took him outside, was he warm enough? Was he allergic to dust—our apartment was so dusty. Was his car seat the safest we could find? Did he get all his shots?

If Roni criticized Asher, my mother was furious, but bit her tongue. When Roni criticized me, however, smoke billowed out of my mom's ears. But her most aggressive response was an oblique reminder to always stick up for myself. Nitpicking was Roni's nature, I explained, but it scratched a raw nerve for my mom because my dad was hypercritical.

My mom traded her two wonderful kids against the lunacy of her marriage. My dad was never home, he brazenly flirted with other women under the pretext that he was an art photographer, he gambled away our Bar Mitzvah money in the stock market, and he refused to socialize with the neighbors, leaving my mom socially isolated. My dad never bought furniture and built our family room couch and chairs in his basement workshop. For nine years the house remained semi-furnished and only half the rooms had been painted. Besides the annual week at the Jersey Shore, we took just one real family vacation in eighteen years. When I was sixteen, my mom asked me if she should divorce him. "But I'm worried about you and Paul," she said. She was guilty about breaking up the home.

"What could be worse than growing up in a house where there is screaming all the time?" I replied. My mother came from a world where people did not split up, but she made a courageous leap and they were finally divorced in the summer of 1978.

My mom was quirky and fun, though. She took Paul and me to drive-ins to see horror and sci-fi double features. We kept lizards and snakes and fed them live mice. She let us have minibikes when we were ten and eleven and bought me *Penthouse* when I was fourteen. During a trip home my freshman year of college, she accidentally washed an entire ounce of marijuana I forgot in my jeans, then left the bag of pot out to dry, and never mentioned it. When she visited my tiny, illegal fifth-floor sublet in New York, she smoked cigarettes in the hallway with my friends Stacey Sherman and Linda Robak. They conspired to fix me up with the right woman. She loved being one of the girls.

My mom came from a working-class home in Trenton, New Jersey. She worked year-round in her mother's orthopedic shoe store, while juggling all the household responsibilities alone. My mother never complained, never raised her voice, and never became angry at anyone, except at my dad, if he yelled at me or my brother.

My mother had simple tastes. She read Sidney Sheldon and Leon Uris novels. We watched *The Night Stalker, Adam-12, The Rookies,* and *Emergency!* She loved to eat at the Seafood Shanty or one of Philadelphia's ramshackle crab houses. Her taste in music leaned toward Barry Manilow, Neil Diamond, and Barbra Streisand.

After three days in the ICU, my mom is moved to a stepdown unit. She lectures me about losing weight. "Don't make the mistakes I made. Take care of your health," she says.

Her recovery is bumpy. I have tense arguments with the obnoxious, blowhard NYU chief resident about her care. My mom has an undiagnosed infection and loses control of her bladder and bowels. They forget to feed her for three days straight. Her arms are black and blue from incompetent blood draws. The cardiac surgeon assures me they anticipated a slow, complicated recovery. Paul flies back to Anchorage and now I juggle the kids, who are sick with winter colds; Agnes; commuting into the city; fighting with the hospital; and managing my mom's recovery.

I tell my mom the hard part is over. She survived the surgery and now everything will be okay. She just has to hang in there, keep her spirits up, eat and sleep and rest. She smiles at me and says she would like an apple muffin. I am worried about how she is really feeling, because I know she will not complain.

On *NYPD Blue*, Bobby Simone goes into NYU Hospital with a heart problem. He dies. "I don't like this show anymore," I tell my mom. "It's too melodramatic."

One night I take the kids to the Food Emporium in the red wagon. Asher is ordered to walk or the wagon will jam in the automatic door. "Why do *I* always have to walk? You never make the *babies* walk," Asher complains. He is at the age where parental ineptitude demands that all his statements be underlined.

Asher understands why I need him to walk a few feet, but emotionally, every sacrifice represents a sleazy legal loophole granted the triplets. I am not in the mood and warn Asher to keep moving, because he is blocking my legs with his body. "They don't have to walk!" Asher insists. "It's not fair."

"Life's not fair," I say, knowing I will regret this, as I regret every other parental cliché—because I said so, I told you so, I don't have to explain this to you, you can make your own rules when you're eighteen. Later, when Asher complains he has to clean up his toys but the triplets don't, I let him watch TV past his bedtime so I can check up on my mom.

On the Saturday three weeks after surgery, my mother's best friend, Ellen, plans to visit for the whole day. My mom is scheduled for an MRI of her stomach and sounds depressed. "I just want everyone to leave me alone," she says. This is unusual for her. I tell her I am sorry and I will be there when Ellen leaves. Ellen is loud and boisterous and wacky and will cheer her up, I hope.

I arrive at the hospital at 5:15 with chicken soup and cold ginger ale. My mom looks exhausted. She doesn't have her blanket on—she runs hot, like me—but when I touch her she is cold. I cover her and hold her hand. She sits up and tries to tell me something, but she is too tired, and slumps back down in the bed.

"That's okay—rest up, Mom, you can tell me later," I say. Her hand is black and blue and swollen up like a baseball. I am feeling really agitated and unsteady. At the nurse's station I ask when the last time her blood pressure and pulse were taken. The nurse on duty doesn't know.

I try talking to my mom, but she isn't responsive. Then she throws up something that looks like coffee grounds. I don't know what to do. I don't know what is wrong. I go to the nurse's station and ask for help. I feel as if I am moving in slow motion. They tell me to wait for the resident making rounds.

After a few minutes I drag the resident out of the hallway. He tries to find my mom's pulse, but is clumsy and moves like molasses. He spends five minutes looking for his stethoscope. I think about dialing 911. One of the ICU nurses said patients sometimes call 911 when the staff is slow.

In fifteen minutes another resident comes in, then another, and then they kick me out behind a shield of whispers, dumping me in a small office.

I realize that I am in shock. I have wasted critical minutes. I should have been in the hallway screaming code blue, code red, whatever they yell on TV. Now I hear people running. A crash cart goes by. I hear voices yelling my mom's name.

Tonight is the second night of Hanukkah. My mom bought Asher a toy cash register for the first night, but Roni had some annoying gift-dispersal conflict. Tonight I will give Asher the cash register. My mom is waiting to hear his reaction.

At about 8:30 I see the snotty chief resident I argued with so many times. He leads me to a small office. The cardiac surgeon is waiting on the phone. The chief resident calls him by his first name, which sounds strange, and hands me the phone. They did everything they could, the cardiac surgeon says, even open-heart massage. They don't know what happened. Her heart looked fine and the grafts were solid. Maybe something toxic got into her system. He is sorry. We could try an autopsy. Sometimes, he says, people in hospitals just die.

FIFTEEN

No Means No (and Other Lies)

The line for coffee at the Hay Day gourmet market stretches down into the baked goods section. The women are angry because this kind of everyday inconvenience mocks their success at marrying so skillfully. I sit at one of the tables, drinking Sumatra and reading *The New York Times*. It is 9:15 A.M. on a Monday morning.

I am the only man in this fishbowl of women who abandoned high-profile careers as lawyers, doctors, bankers, and public-relations executives to stay at home and manage the kids. It is somewhat frightening to see these supermoms channel their hyperaggressive personalities into renovating, decorating, overseeing the household staff and relentless play-date organizing. I keep my head down and drink my coffee.

One of the moms knows me from Asher's after-school program and asks about the family. We moved out of Bronxville and into Scarsdale at the end of August, I explain, right before kindergarten started for Asher.

It is November 1999. The triplets are almost three years old now. They attend nursery school at a local synagogue in the morning and a Montessori school in the afternoon.

"Oh," the woman says. "So you . . . stay at home?"

Yes, I say. I am a stay-at-home dad. For almost a year now.

Mikimoto pearls jangle against bony necks as heads turn my way. The only men visible during the day in Scarsdale are contractors, deliverymen, and Wall Street shysters serving out the house-arrest portion of their sentences. I am an anomaly, like a mermaid or an anarchist.

"I think that's great," the woman says. "I wish my husband spent more time home with the kids. He goes in to the office on the third day of a three-day weekend because he goes crazy being locked up with the kids."

I hear that story a lot, I say, editing out my opinion that it is nonsense. If these women wanted husbands who spent more time home with the kids, they would marry carpenters or painters or chemistry teachers and live upstate in New Paltz or Peekskill or Oneonta, where they would shop at Wal-Mart and buy day-old bread at the outlet store and muddle by with three unrenovated bedrooms and one and a half baths. If any one of these plastic surgeons or investment bankers or personal injury lawyers told his wife he was taking a year off to study metal sculpture and drive the soccer carpool and create balance in his life, he would have more lawyers in his house than O.J. Simpson.

It is 9:45 now. I fold up my newspaper and go home. My coffee break lasts exactly thirty minutes, the amount of time I would spend on the train into the city.

.   .   .

The stay-at-home dad, a popular trend story in magazines and Sunday newspapers, is a socially awkward reality in the suburbs, the most reactionary social environment in America. In cities like Austin or St. Paul or San Francisco, we would just be another quirky couple. But in a suburb like ours the other dads look at me with a confusion that borders on fear, and the moms, while boosterish in their enthusiasm for our alternative lifestyle, are unable to absorb me into their viciously organized social circles.

Roni suffers the most, since working moms occupy the lowest rung on the social ladder (the sole exception being the stay-at-home dad). Moms who work suffer at the hands of an apartheid apparatus that is all the more oppressive because it is so transparent. Power begins with the Class Moms and radiates outward in a fiendishly calibrated spiral of social engineering, gossiping, and backstabbing. Hysteria and paranoid delusions are traded over morning coffee and low-fat scones. One of the moms in our neighborhood became obsessed by the fear that her three-year-old son's penis was smaller than normal, so she lobbied the other moms to let her examine the competitive field artillery to determine if she was outgunned. Normally, this kind of behavior would spell the end for a family's reputation, but this mom was thin and attractive and friendly enough to pull it off. In this way the suburbs are like ninth grade.

Roni and I both grew up in row houses in working-class neighborhoods—Roni in Queens, me in Northwest Philadelphia. She loathes the materialism and high school cliquishness and mindless home-decorating chitchat and would leave in a heartbeat for some small town in Vermont or New Mexico or Upstate New York. Sometimes she scrolls through on-line real estate listings around the country and calls me over to tell me how much house we could get for $180,000 if only we packed up our stuff and ran away. No more treading water, no more stacks of unpaid medical bills, no more shutoff notices from the cable TV company and cell phone provider.

"Let's buy a Winnebago and drive around the country," Roni says one morning, apropos of nothing, when the kids are screaming around the kitchen, not listening to our demands that they put their shoes on so we can leave the house.

"That was always my dad's big dream," I say.

A cold shiver runs up my spine as I consider the circumlocution of the weirdness gene. I grew up in an unpainted suburban house and my amateur photographer dad took nude pictures of women in an empty upstairs bedroom when he wasn't in the basement yelling at my brother and me to be quiet and stop running around the house. Even though I joke about it, the parallels between Roni and my dad are a bit frightening. They both love hardware stores, power tools, and construction sites. They both love to take pictures and fiddle around in a darkroom. They are both infatuated with bargains and will spend hours to save a few dollars. They both tend to be autocratic and immune to self-analysis, although my father is much more extreme.

The scariest similarity, though, is that both Roni and my dad have the habit of starting projects they never finish, along with the inability to see this character trait. My brother and I grew up in a home with no furniture and unpainted rooms. My dad built a couch and two chairs out of hardwood in the basement when I was a teenager, but he never finished or stained them. The furniture remained in this state of limbo in our living room for years and, after the divorce, moved with my dad into his tumbledown row house, where they remain still happily united—and still unfinished—today, more than thirty years later. Our new house in Scarsdale is filled with temporary, thrift-store furniture because Roni tends to juggle eight or ten decorating projects at a time, unable to finish off any single room. Roni built our first bed from scratch when we lived in the city—and it's beautiful—but never stained or finished it. It has traveled with us to Bronxville and now to Scarsdale, where, ten years later, it is the center of a guest bedroom, still unfinished and unpainted. The bed is a ghost from my past—the ghost of unfinished business—that only I can see.

It took me a long time to understand that part of our connection is that Roni and I both grew up in weird homes. Roni grew up speaking German and Czech and Hungarian and ate fried pork fat and her parents had no friends. Now our kids are growing up in the Mr. Mom-and-Mrs. Lawyer house. To lean into the weirdness even harder, the kids have different last names: Two are Stocklers and two are Fischers. Long before Roni and I were married, she made me promise that when we had kids, we would split up the last names, because both sides of her family were wiped out in World War II. It was an abstraction, so I said yes. But when people learn the kids have alternating last names they look at us as if we are unbalanced. Even the woman in the hospital administration office looked at me sideways when I filled out the birth certificates. One of my old college buddies, Howard Katz, told me I was going to ruin their lives.

One day in the elementary school parking lot, Liza, one of the friendliest, most down-to-earth of the moms, asks if I want to join her weekly book-reading club. I burst out laughing. "That would be the end for me," I explain. Roni could tolerate my taking up a kinky afternoon sex club or robbing a bank, but sitting around in ladies' living rooms discussing literature would be the marital coup de grâce.

To forestall criticism from the late-at-work mom, the stay-at-home dad tries to create motivational systems, implementation methodologies, and psychological profiling techniques to organize the children's daily routine. The children have better ideas.

The stay-at-home dad's day begins at 6:30 A.M., when Jared wakes up. Jared is the most physically attuned of the brood and puts himself to bed, even during a favorite cartoon, when tired.

By 7:30 the last child is awake and the getting-dressed game begins. In the rules of this game, the TV is turned on and off, like a morphine drip, to motivate children to dress. The late-at-work mom suggests not paying the cable bill.

Hannah and Jared normally dress without incident. Asher requires repeated warnings and threatened removal of privileges, while Barak extorts adult assistance by filibustering—lying on his side, sucking his thumb, clutching his yellow blanket. When the stay-at-home dad attempts to put on Barak's clothes, he flops around on the ground like a boneless chicken.

Breakfast begins at 8:05 to 8:10. On any given day the kids may quietly eat a bowl or two of cereal or descend into Balkanized fighting. Some days the stay-at-home dad counts to ten and separates the children. Some days he starts laughing out of nervous excitement and lets entropy work its course. And some days he screams at them to quiet down, which is counterproductive, because screaming only begets more screaming. Asher's lunch is made, backpacks packed, coats laid out, teeth brushed.

The battle over leaving then ensues. This battle pits inertia against momentum. Children instructed to sit on the couch with their shoes develop time-devouring problems elsewhere. Asher is upstairs searching for a library book. Barak sits on the couch with one sock and no shoes. Jared wears one sneaker and dismantles a toy that may or may not belong to Barak but which provokes howls of protest. Hannah actually puts on her shoes and ties them, unassisted.

Inertia demands that the stay-at-home dad forget critical tasks, such as note signing and club paying and conference scheduling. The stay-at-home dad dashes upstairs for the checkbook and returns to find Asher playing the electronic piano, Barak clomping around in Roni's high heels, Jared MIA, Hannah screaming.

The house is locked, backpacks, hats, and gloves double-checked. The Suburban is opened and children given a three-count. The kids fight over air rights for climbing over seats. The detours are legion, like the names of Noah's family running across Genesis.

The stay-at-home dad drives to Asher's elementary school and walks Asher to his first grade class. The triplets are driven to the reformed temple in New Rochelle.

The stay-at-home dad works on his freelance writing assignments until 11:15, makes lunch, and dashes back to the temple at 11:45. The triplets have thirty minutes to eat in a lounge that has couches and tables, usually with a few other children and their stay-at-home moms. The stay-at-home dad is cordial to the stay-at-home moms, even as he visualizes his testicles floating in a jar on his wife's desk.

The kids run across the couches in the lounge, even though the purpose of couches for sitting has been explained 37,000 times. Jared shares important information about the teachers and class projects, Hannah explains the emotional ups and downs of the children, and Barak spins elaborate fantasy scenarios about friends, dogs, flying saucers, crabs, and talking marshmallows.

At 1:15 the kids are driven from the synagogue to the local Montessori school, where their habitual lateness is a source of amusement for the warm and generous staff. The stay-at-home dad works on his articles from 1:45 until 2:45, not counting errands and phone calls. The triplets are picked up at 3:00.

Between 3:15 and 5:30 the stay-at-home dad supervises multiple activities, handles minor emergencies, preps dinner, and tries to reduce the state of physical bedlam in the house to a state of clutter. At 6:30 the children are packed in the car and driven to pick up Asher, whose full-day schedule promotes his independence.

At 7:00 P.M. dinner is prepared. The stay-at-home dad is conned into preparing four completely separate meals, in direct violation of the late-at-work mom's one-meal-only food-service philosophy.

After dinner and cleanup and the unpacking of backpacks and inventorying of lost hats and gloves comes the donning of PJs, the starting of laundry, the reading of books, and the watching of TV. This is the bridge to bedtime, a nightly battle for one more show, fifteen more minutes, one more minute, just one, anything for one more minute of blessed and sustaining TV.

The late-at-work wife returns home between 9:00 and 10:00, exhausted and dispirited, horrified by one or more errors of the stay-at-home dad (the garbage! the recycling! the Tupperware!), who is delighted to hear his domestic shortcomings read back to him.

The stay-at-home dad juggles the intersecting trajectories of his family's days—the kids as they fight off the unfair sentence of sleep, and the late-at-work mom, who wants hugs and kisses from the kids but, more than anything, mental decompression time. More chores—adult laundry, straightening up, sweeping, cooking adult dinner, garbage bagged—are layered into the simmering riot of late evening. The stay-at-home dad serves dinner and brings the late-at-work mom a treat as she falls asleep on the couch, struggling to make it through *All My Children*.

At 11:00 P.M. Barak is taken to pee in his sleep, pots and dishes cleaned, the dishwasher loaded, garbage taken outside, kitchen floors vacuumed, lights turned off, house locked. At 11:30 or 12:00 the stay-at-home dad writes for an hour if he is lucky and ambitious. At 12:30 or 1:15 A.M. he retucks the kids in their beds, turns down the heat, double-checks the house, and watches TV.

At 1:30 or 2:00 A.M. the stay-at-home dad climbs into bed, only to wake again at 4:00 or 5:00 to take a child to the potty, fetch someone a drink of water, soothe the victim of a nightmare. Out of the darkness a heavy weight attacks the stay-at-home dad's chest. Is he dreaming of a heart attack? Or is he waking to a major biological event?

Jared kneels on the stay-at-home dad's chest and squeezes his face with his strong hands.

"Daddy?" Jared says. The clock reads 6:18.

"Yes, Jared? says the stay-at-home dad.

"Can we play a game?" Jared says.

The kids run from room to room, naked (in the new house, in Scarsdale, all the bedrooms connect) as I prepare their every-other-day bath. (The exhaustion of bathing four kids at the end of a long day trumps my embarrassment at cutting corners with their personal hygiene.) They disobey every order—to put their clothes in the hamper, stop running, go potty, stop flying off the chairs.

"Hannah, come," commands Jared, from the TV room.

"Whatwhatwhat?" Hannah says, annoyed. This is new, this sense that when her mind is occupied her brothers trespass in speaking to her.

I don't hear the words, but they are conspiring. I hear feet clomping and then see the smiling face of Barak. He smiles overenthusiastically at me, coincidentally holding his penis and testicles and scrunching them up in the air like a ball of Play-Do. My explanation that a person's private parts are not toys is generally ignored.

"Daddy! Whatcha doing in there!" Barak says, feigning surprise at finding me. He is a scout sent forward to collect intelligence. He runs away, stopping to bend over and waggle his tushie at me.

"Guys! Guys!" Rocky yells. I hear the superheated whispering, the interrupting, bragging, nonsense, singing, sound effects, whining, banging, the noisy radio traffic.

Asher and the triplets have grown exceptionally closer over the last year. Identical twins often develop a private, nonverbal language, but these three are hyperverbal and compete to make themselves seen, felt, heard, and understood. With Asher, they launch schemes and counterschemes against me, conspire toward some mundane end, and then suddenly dissolve their alliance in bitter fighting, scratching, hurt feelings, and angry accusations.

The growing emotional closeness of the four children is due, in large part, to the new sleeping arrangements. In the Scarsdale house, all four kids sleep together in one bedroom, as in a military barracks. This was Roni's scheme to help them bond and to keep Asher integrated. I was bitterly opposed to this at first because Asher loved his bedroom in the Bronxville house, but now I see the genius behind the move. The triplets were babies in the old house and Asher needed his privacy. Now they are closer developmentally and the four of them are bonding like crazy. They share books and toys and root around in one another's special boxes. Most of all, they band together to defy parental authority after they are given their last lights-out warning, at which point they turn into a rebel army—they turn the lights back on, play games, goof around, leap from bed to bed, trade toys and pillows and blankets, fight and make up and regroup. We build an extra half-hour into bedtime to let them blow off steam together.

After I put the kids in bed and close the security gate, I stand in the hallway and eavesdrop. Asher launches some complicated plan to bilk them out of their toys or attempts some ill-fated attack that will leave them holding the bag. Jared and Hannah discuss their stuffed doggies' agendas for the night. Barak spouts a barrage of words, a nonstop channeling of some private toddler meta-text.

The kids exchange delicate observations about Roni and me as if lifted from CIA surveillance tapes. I hear bizarre question-and-answer sessions—"Does the summer have a birthday?"—vicious taunting, sudden outbursts of off-key singing and yodeling. Asher unleashes some furious explanation to debunk an innocent piece of misinformation offered by one of the triplets. Once in a while Barak or Hannah suddenly says, "Oh, fuck it!" or "Goddamn it!" in pitch-perfect imitation of me, followed by Asher's intentionally pompous sentencing of time-out, his impersonation of me a bombastic, white-wigged English barrister.

Now the triplets are missing, in the middle of a covert op. They scaled the security gate—Jared, the acrobat, taught them how—and snuck downstairs. I hear them search for cookies as a metal tin clatters to the ground.

"Not that one!" shouts Hannah.

"I know, I know!" Jared says.

"I'm going shlooping in your bed," Barak sings.

"Stop it!" Hannah yells.

"Schlooping nopping habba-nabba looping ko ko ko jopping," Barak adds, stoking Hannah's misplaced fury.

"I think it's brok-en," Jared says, enunciating for emphasis. "Let's put it back."

"Yaaaaaargh!" I hear. Asher was reading his book, but the chance to launch a surprise ambush on the triplets was too tantalizing to ignore.

Four kids bellow jolt trip boil elbow clang up the steps like an army. The triplets scream the fur out of their lungs as Asher chases them, whipping them ahead with a cheap plastic sword.

The babies take the turn into the hallway at full speed,

even as I yell at them to stop. Asher smacks Barak, who pushes Jared, who bangs his head on the wall and crumples to the floor like a brown paper bag.

"Stop!" I scream. *"Stooooopppp!"*

Jared bawls furiously as I scoop him up. Asher chases Barak and Hannah through the connecting bedrooms and emerges from the master bedroom to crash into my legs. Asher pinballs away but I grab him by the arm, hard.

"I said stop!" I yell, holding him by the arm.

"But Daddy, we're playing," Asher says, innocently.

Barak pulls on my arm, jamming his fingers into my thumb, trying to free Asher. "Guys! Guys! The bad Daddy got Asher, help, help," Barak says. "Get off, Daddy!"

Asher pulls on my arm. "Come on, Daddy!" he says.

"No means no," I say. "Don't move." When I readjust Jared on my shoulder, Asher and Barak bolt with Hannah in tow. They ignore me as I yell, threaten, and remove privileges. I put Jared down and when they cycle through the bedroom again I grab Asher and Barak, spin them around, and whack them on their naked bottoms once each with my open hand. I whip the plastic sword into the closet and slam the door shut.

"I said no more!" I scream. *"No means no! What don't you understand about the word 'no'!"*

"Ow, ow, ow!" Barak screams, holding his bottom. Asher is crying too. "You're so mean, *I hate you!*" Asher says. He runs into the bedroom, climbs into his bed, and hides his face in his hands.

"You'resomeansmellybaddaddydon'tlistentomeworstdaddyIdidn'tdoanythingyoudon'tknowwhatyou'retalking!" Barak rants. Tears pour down his face and I feel like shit.

The past year has been a hard one for me. I don't enforce time-outs consistently. I count to three and then count again. I stick them in time-out and they escape without consequence. During multiple time-outs, they rumble and carry on like prison gangs. It's grueling to juggle three or four simultaneous time-outs and I need an Excel spreadsheet to track the matrix of lost privileges. They exploit and overwhelm the weaknesses in the criminal justice system, which makes me angry, even though it's my own fault.

I hug Barak and tell him I love him. He resists at first, but I am good at this job, even if not much else. Barak punches me in the chest, hard. He enjoys wearing high heels and plastic necklaces, but the boy packs a wallop.

"Ow," I say. Barak pulls his head back. His freckly, blond-haired face is red from crying, but his mischievous smile is poking through. He punches me again.

"Ow!" I say.

"Kill him!" Asher says from the bedroom.

"I'm going to cut your neck off," Barak says, narrowing his eyes into an evil stare. Barak makes a sawing motion with his hand. Cutting people's necks off is one of his new preoccupations.

"Asher," I say. "That's not nice."

"You're not nice," Asher says.

"I'm sorry I yelled at you, and I'm sorry I hit you," I say to Asher. "But you guys were out of control. You need to listen when I say no."

Barak is sawing my head off and cackling with appreciation.

"Apology . . . not accepted!" Asher declares. He holds up his arm and points to the door. "Just because you're mad at Mommy doesn't mean you can be mean to us."

I sit quietly and look at my boy. Roni called while I was serving the kids dinner to complain I hadn't paid her Visa bill, one thing led to another, and I went upstairs to my office so the kids wouldn't hear us trade accusations.

"You're right," I tell Asher. "I shouldn't get mad at you because I'm mad at Mommy." I can only imagine the depth his observations will reach by the time he is fifteen.

It has been a long year for me, if you accept that some years may be longer than others. I have anger issues. I am angry at myself for not seeing how my mom's recovery was going wrong and not ordering an independent autopsy. I am angry at the hospital for a number of unresolved issues, such as why I was never told my mom's infection was serious, and that she had been moved up to the "last chance" antibiotic. I am angry at Roni for expecting me to put this all behind me. I am angry at the pinch-faced old ladies in line at the gourmet market, complaining about the produce, for living so long when my mother did not.

The timing was bad for a major decision, but we decided to buy a house in Scarsdale. I needed a distraction and the Bronxville house held too many painful reminders of how much I had taken my mom for granted.

We found a large fixer-upper that needed serious TLC. I worked on the house every day for a month. I ripped out moldy old wall-to-wall carpets and scraped up the forty-year-old carpet backing, which dissolved like broken Cheez-It crackers. With a hammer I knocked out built-in closets. I painted and hammered and sawed. It felt good to work with my hands, to work twelve hour days with no lunch break and no talking. I tore out trees and dug down a mysterious mound in the backyard to flatten and square off the property. One day three fingers on my right hand went numb. I ignored the pain for a week but it only grew worse. I was diagnosed with carpal tunnel syndrome and needed surgery on both hands. I told the doctors to do the right hand and wait on the left. I didn't want to spend any more time in hospitals than absolutely necessary.

The house was like us—quirky, comfortable, messy, and modest. The house needed so much work that I sometimes imagined it wanted to see me buried in the backyard, but the kids loved it and saw none of the flaws. The rooms connected on the second floor in a grand prix loop and there were endless closets and attic rooms to hide in. They tore around the yard and up and down the driveway. They chased birds and bunny rabbits and squirrels and chipmunks.

I sneak into the kids' bedroom after they are asleep and straighten out their covers. Barak is still awake and smiles up at me.

"Grandma's in heaven, right, Daddy?" Barak says. The kids ask about her out of the blue. On the nights I am thinking about my mom, I wonder what this coincidence means.

"That's right," I say. Better to grow up with the comfort. Einstein believed.

Barak smiles and hugs my arm and makes his special little ooey-gooey sounds. I wrap his yellow blanket around him. My mom barely knew the triplets. They were twenty-two months old when she died, and will not remember her.

Mom would be mad at you for yelling at the kids, I say to myself. She never, ever yelled. Dad yelled. The only thing I ever knew about fatherhood was that I would not yell. I would not be like my dad.

Don't yell at the kids now. You've failed enough. Don't break this one promise.

I look at the picture Asher drew in blue pencil for my mom when she was in the hospital. I peeled it off the hospital wall the night she died, brought it home, and hung it on the wall of my home office. For the first time, I notice there are seven crudely drawn pencil figures—Asher has many talents, but drawing is not among them—and wonder if the seventh figure is supposed to be my mom, standing with the six of us, watching over us, as she promised me the morning before her surgery.

My mother would be so proud of Asher. He is so warm and loving and funny and sensitive. A month or so after she died, we were at a shopping mall play zone for kids. The triplets were bouncing and running and screaming, and I sat off in a corner, staring into space and thinking regretfully about my mom. Out of the blue, Asher snuck up next to me and said, "Are you thinking about Grandma?" He was four years old.

It comforts me to realize that I love my children fiercely because I was so fiercely loved. This was my mother's gift. I don't remember if I ever told her as much, or if she saw inside me her own enormous strength. But this becomes my myth: My mom will live on, in this randomly ordered universe, through me, as I love my kids above all.

SIXTEEN

In the Ladies' Room

I am in the ladies' room.

It is filled with ladies—old ladies, working ladies, teenage ladies, and young ladies-in-training. And me—a goateed, balding, moderately overweight man of forty.

"I'm sorry," I say. This is a generalized gender-to-gender apology. I keep my eyes averted, my head down, a bathroom-crashing penitent.

Who is in charge here? Is there a head lady?

I pat the heads of my kids. "Men's room, disgusting, the toilet, I have four," I say. It is late December, and the triplets are a month shy of their third birthday.

"Daddy!" Asher says. "Close the door!" Asher wants me to step inside the stall where he is conducting his business. I look down and take a head count. One, two, three.

Three? Three is not good. Three means one is missing. I began with four, of that fact I am sure. We are in a massive shopping mall in a small town outside Albany, in Upstate New York, during a visit to my in-laws. I don't understand how an economically depressed area can support a huge mall boasting luxury stores. The large sodas in the movie theater cost $5.50, more than Manhattan. Something is strange here. This is neither the time nor the place to lose 25 percent of my kids.

I call out Barak's name.

"Daddy, close the door and come inside," Asher whines.

I explain that I can't leave the triplets alone as Jared and Hannah perform the pee-pee dance. They do not appreciate delays in the potty traffic control system.

The triplets are competitive. As a group they compete against their older brother for time, attention, food, the good chairs in the TV room. They compete individually for toys, favors, portion control, love. Between one another they struggle in dense, furtive ways that still elude me. I'm not sure what branch of mathematics is required to diagram the vectors of all this competition. I do know that watching one of your siblings find relief in the bathroom magnifies your own needs many times over.

"I have to make a poopie!" whines Hannah. She pats her rear end for dramatic emphasis.

"Where's Rocky?" I ask Asher, who sits on the toilet, head in his hand. He looks up, red-faced and tired. It has been a long day. Something has upset his stomach.

"He was right there," Asher says, gesturing inconclusively. The natural vagueness of his gesture increases my anxiety. I don't see or hear Barak at all. "I have to go—"

"No, Daddy!" Asher shouts, his face screwing up into a mask of anxiety. He grabs my arm. Despite his confidence he still sometimes shifts into a clammy fear of abandonment. "Don't leave me!" he pleads.

"Daddy!" Hannah yells. She is trying to open the stall

next to Asher's, which is occupied, by a lady.

"Hannah!" I say.

"Excuse me," says a lady's voice from inside the stall.

"Barak!" I yell. Condescending glares baste me in bad ladies' karma.

I am competitive, too, ladies, so stand back. Who among you has changed fourteen thousand diapers? Can any one of you catch pizza-and-grape-juice vomit in her arms and heave it out a taxicab window at thirty miles an hour? None of you can carry three whimpering thirty-pound kids up a flight of stairs simultaneously while sustaining a flurry of testicle-hammering kicks. I haven't lost my son . . . exactly. He's hiding somewhere within the sound of my voice. I know my kids as well as I know myself, or even better.

Ten minutes before, the kids and I are riding up and down the escalators. The escalators are the closest my family will come to Disneyland, at least for a few years. They shriek with delight as we go up and down again and again. Up the escalator, down the escalator. Up and down. They whoop with happiness. Ironically, this activity is completely free.

The triplets are two years and eleven months old now. They are just out of diapers, thanks to Roni's hard work and Asher's elevating influence. It is December, the week of Hanukkah, and we are visiting Roni's parents. I need to take the kids out and exercise them and burn up some discontent and the mall is perfect because they can run, explore, and express themselves at full volume. December is a hard month for me, the week of Hanukkah especially. How unfair that such a beautiful holiday now symbolizes death for me, and the pleasure of giving gifts to my kids is eaten away by regret and self-recrimination. I could have done so much more to help my mom. So I like to stay busy. The mall is good. The mall is busy, I am busy watching them cavort, and they are whoopingly happy. It is a good afternoon.

"Hi, mans," Hannah says to a gangly man on the down escalator.

"Nyah-uh, nyah-uh, nyah-uh," sings Barak, gyrating in place. Rocky loves the escalators the most. He tries to climb the handrail, squirm out of my grip. He squeals with joy as pure as Viennese marzipan.

We are having fun. We are going up, we are going down. We have a full supply of provisions, soft pretzels and lemonade, sold by brusque, nose-ringed teenagers.

"I need to go potty," Asher says.

"Are you sure?" I say.

"Daddy," he says. For a moment, I forget he is the child and I am the father.

The one problem with toilet training children is that freedom from diapers creates the burden of always remaining within striking distance of a bathroom. I maintain a hyperawareness of the nearest toilet. I am an organic-based potty global positioning system, constantly recalculating my status vis-à-vis children's services. We are now in the period where child care is actually more work than the previous stage of development, the poopie amendment to the law of unintended consequences.

Barak must be carried away from the escalators, screaming, feet kicking. I promise him a return trip, treats, extra TV. Like Asher, Barak has a hard time with transitions. The four of us study the mall legend, even though I don't know why malls bother with them. According to the schematic, the nearest bathroom is located in a vertical crawl space behind a hidden tunnel that leads to a portal into the fourth dimension.

Fifteen minutes later we find the men's room and my worst fears are realized. One stall, one urinal, one sink.

"Fu—" I start to say.

Asher opens the stall door and walks in. His pants drop to the ground.

"Wait!" I scream.

I carry him out of the stall. "Forget it," I say. "We're not staying here!"

The bathroom is bad. Not bad like a sloppy college roommate, but bad like the Middle Ages.

"But Daddy, I have to *go!*" Asher says. I drag my contingent into the hallway, frantic now. I am angry. I pay some of the highest state taxes in the country, vote, and place my litter in the garbage. I deserve a clean, well-lit place to take my children to the bathroom.

What am I going to do? Run the kids across the mall, crying and wailing? Bribe my way into the Pizza 'N' Brew three levels up?

Then I see the ladies' room.

No, I think. It is not done. I am Man. Destroyer of worlds. Spoiler of tropical climates. Eater of soups.

Even that word—*ladies*—frightens me. My wife wears work boots and flannel shirts around the house. My women friends matched me tequila shot for tequila shot back in my single days. "Ladies" are scary, alien creatures who wear red blazers and silk stockings and waltz into Bergdorf's with high expectations and Amex cards.

"Daddy, I have to go!" Asher says.

"I have to go, too!" announces Hannah.

"Me, too!" says Barak.

Jared smiles up at me. "I have to make a poopie," he says, traitorously.

Potty training has made the kids' intestinal itineraries align weirdly, the way college women in dorms menstruate in unison. Some crazy pee-pee mojo soldiers on out there, and when one kid has to go, they all need to go, even if they don't.

I peer into the ladies' room, my blood pressure clenching upward. It is shiny and clean. Ladies' rooms are almost always clean. And it is here. It is full of ladies, of course, a real obstacle. Or is it? Maybe the obstacle is just in my mind.

I make an executive decision. We are going in.

"We can't go in here!" says Asher. "It's for *girls!*"

I keep my eyes glued to the floor, as if this might somehow provide a cloak of invisibility. Asher hops up and down while I begin my cumbersome public-restroom-cleansing ritual. I wet paper towels with warm water and wash the toilet seat and bowl, then lift up the seat and clean along the whole inside rim.

Then I clean the front and sides of the toilet bowl, where Asher's legs hang down, and then the floor. I discard the paper towels, dry the seat carefully, throw away this second set of towels, and wash my hands.

As a child, I had vivid, recurring nightmares in which I ran away from a faceless monster that caught my neck or cheek with razor-sharp hooks and then tore off huge sections of my face flesh—too much occult and horror story reading material. In my nightmares now I am trapped in filthy men's rooms with my kids and there are no paper towels. My adult nightmare comes true on a regular basis.

I try to shove basketball-sized wads of wet paper towels into the constricted waste chute, but they do not fit. The bathroom is trying to jam me up, but, mentally, I am moving at the speed of light. I am Antibacterial Man.

"Daddy!" Asher yells. He considers my frantic scrubbing deranged. Finally, I put him on the seat.

"Daddy, I have to go!" Hannah says, pulling her dress up to her neck.

Out of the corner of my eye, I see a security guard glaring at me from the hallway. "Everything okay in there?" the security guard says. He is large, with a shaven head. Evidently, though, he lacks the will to set foot in a ladies' room full of ladies.

I hold my breath. None of the ladies say anything. Maybe they are jaded by movies and cable television, where a man in the ladies' room is just another quirk of modern life. Maybe there was a man in the ladies' room on *Friends*.

Secretly I enjoy forcing my way into the ladies' room. I have always been fascinated by ladies' rooms. But I am disappointed. No abstract Georgia O'Keeffe-y interpretations of female genitalia on the walls. No Uma Thurmanish ladies slouch around on distressed leather couches, smoking cigarettes, reading *Vanity Fair*.

Aside from the number of toilet seats and overall cleanliness, the ladies' room turns out to be a mundane parallel of the men's room. Despite the difference in age, size and social status, the ladies all busy themselves with various self-enhancement regimens. The ladies spray on waves of perfume, polish their nails, apply makeup or makeup remover, lacquer their hair with hair spray.

Now I know the real reason smoking is forbidden in ladies' rooms—to prevent ladies from exploding.

A sandy blond head pokes in from the outside hallway, Barak's demented, puppet-show, Harpo Marx entrance.

"I'm in the hallway, oh-sticky Daddy-hey," Barak sings. He dances across the threshold to the room, throwing little disco gestures at me, laughing out loud at his own ineffable behavior.

"I have to goooooo!" Hannah says, stamping her feet.

The stall to our left is still occupied. The stall door to the right opens the wrong way, blocking visual contact inside Asher's stall. Plus, opening a second front means more cleaning and disinfecting.

I am caught between two powerful, negative energies—the objective reality of the stalls' filthiness and my irrational anxiety about public restrooms.

A normal adult sees a highway rest stop as a safe and convenient amenity, but I see a level 5 biohazard. I see men in white space suits and Michael Crichton novels. A life-threatening emergency is the only reason I will sit down in a men's room. Even then, it takes me fifteen minutes to prepare my journey. I lift the seat with my foot, wash the seat and front of the bowl front (where my pants will make contact), wash my hands to cleanse the germs from all this preparation, then create a thick paper barrier on which to perch. To perform the actual touchdown requires several slow and laborious attempts. There may be trouble with the landing gear or disturbances on the ground.

The desecrated state of men's rooms is proof alone that women are biologically and intellectually superior to men.

Asher takes his time and I grow more nervous. A clock is ticking. I fold toilet paper squares for Asher, trying to hurry him along through telekinesis, as Hannah whines more and more urgently.

"You have doggies on your shirt, yeah, you do," Barak sings, to a perplexed girl of fourteen. The girl ignores him and hurries out of the bathroom with her girlfriend. Barak does dance steps in her wake, oblivious to the snub. I am proud of him. Let him carry his insouciance into adulthood and avoid the pain of female indifference.

Jared does pull-ups between two sink basins. Then he leaps up into a push-up, arms extended and locked. He brings his legs up into a crunch and grins at me. He will be the first Stockler in hundreds of years to have six-pack abs.

"Please, Asher," I say. But what is a kid to do? What can I say to hurry him along? I take my own sweet time in the bathroom with at least one section of *The New York Times*. With four kids, my bathroom hiatus represents my only private time between 6:00 A.M. and 10:00 P.M.

Asher finishes and Jared tries to enter the stall. "My turn," he says.

Hannah lets out a scream that sends toilet seats slamming.

"Jared," I beg, kneeling down. I promise him anything—

treats, toys, staying up until midnight. Anything.

Jared has the most physical control of the triplets. His body operates with almost supernatural efficiency, right down to his bowel movements.

"Uppie," Jared says. I am in luck. He will trade an uppie for a potty. Although the obvious future jock, Jared is the most clingy. I feel guilty that he didn't negotiate a better deal, and vow to make it up to him later.

While I pull Hannah up on the seat, Barak drags a yellow Warning! Wet Floor! sign around and sings happily. I ask him to put down the sign.

"You put yourself down," Rocky sings in one of his weird voices. If he were a year older, this would be back talk. For him, it is simply wordplay.

Jared hangs on my neck, pretending he is on the edge of a cliff. I feel Jared balancing his weight, testing himself.

Fifteen minutes click by, slow as a root canal, but Hannah is not ready.

"Hannah," I say. "We have to get out of here." The bathroom grows more and more crowded, as if a movie has just let out.

"Five more poopies coming out," Hannah says. Hannah attaches numerical estimates to all of her toilet business. "I'm making fifty-six poopies now," she'll say. She is by far the most fascinated with her bodily functions.

"I'm going to make a big, smelly poopie," Hannah will say. "Stinky, just for you, Daddy." If Roni is around to hear this, she reacts with terror.

"That's your side of the family," Roni says, eyes narrow

with anger, as though I exert some control over the effect of my DNA.

Roni, meanwhile, is leisurely returning pairs of children's shoes she bought yesterday. Her newest shopping strategy is to buy items we might possibly need and return the ones we don't. She brings home nine pairs of kids' shoes, takes back six. She is building a personalized home shopping network.

So I am trapped in the ladies' room with four kids, and she is out, free and unworried, drinking a latte and gossiping with her older sister, Ruthie.

I am losing my patience. "Let's go," I say.

"Noooo!" Hannah says.

"We have to leave," I say. "We're in the ladies' room!"

Is Hannah doing this on purpose, humiliating me, inconveniencing her brothers, exacting some weird form of control?

"Let's get a cookie," I try. "A PowerPuff Girl toy. Whatever you want."

But Hannah is not budging. She is as stubborn as a mule—her mother's side of the family. Like Asher and me, she also has the sitting-down curse. Barak and Jared have been spared.

I move the three boys out into the hallway. There is no door and we look right into Hannah's stall. "Daddy!" Hannah cries. She reaches out her little arms.

"No. It's time to go," I say. I put on my cold face, my determined face, my assuming-control-of-the-situation face. It is buried deep in the attic.

"Daddy, she needs more time," says Asher, hands on hips, scolding. I am amazed at his ability to switch to counselor and advocate for the triplets.

Roni insists that I be more sympathetic to Hannah's bathroom eccentricities. Hannah has penis envy, she warns. Issues.

She is right. At the playground the boys will stand next to a tree, bare-assed, pants around their ankles, peeing and singing.

"Make a picture!" Asher will say.

"Make circles!" Barak will shout, his little tushie rotating in the air.

Poor Hannah will look up at me, tears cascading down her face. "I want to make pee-pee outside!" she'll say, tugging sadly at the waistband of her shorts. We tried it once. I sacrificed a good pair of New Balance shoes.

Ladies' revenge, I think. We were scheduled to meet Roni in front of Macy's twenty minutes ago. She'll never find us. She watches all the PBS mysteries yet lacks the deductive ability to track us down. What worries me even more is that she will forget about us, drive back to her sister's house, and fall asleep watching TV.

"Daddy, poopie is coming down," Jared says.

I tell Asher to stay in the corridor with Barak where I can see them.

"Come on, Hannah," I say. "It's Jared's turn."

"*No!*" Hannah says.

Jared looks at me. Why don't I do something? "Women," I say.

Five minutes later, I have cleaned the stall next to Hannah and deposited Jared. Now I am getting looks from the ladies—two stalls?

"Daddy, don't leave," Jared says, squeezing my hand.

"I have to check on Hannah," I say.

"Daddy!" Hannah yells from the adjoining stall.

"I'm right here," I say.

"Daddy!" Jared moans.

"Please stop saying 'Daddy'!" I say.

A low point has been reached. You think you're at a low point, and then you discover you were mistaken, the victim of an overly optimistic assessment.

Jared finishes his business in forty-five seconds flat. I walk him into the hallway, go back to offer Hannah more elaborate bribes, and hear the sound of scampering feet. Asher is leading Jared and Rocky down the interlocking corridors used by the maintenance staff. I try to head them off before they explode out into the shopping mall. Hannah screams behind me.

I drag the boys back from an assault on a boiler room door to find the confusing image of Hannah letting a strange woman wipe her rear end.

What to do? Tackle her? Call the police?

The woman smiles warmly. She is in her early thirties, thin, either Indian or Pakistani by her facial features and colorful clothing. Hannah pulls up her stockings and gives me a happy little wave. The incident is more astonishing given that Hannah is extremely suspicious of strange women. It takes Hannah six to eight weeks before she will allow a new baby-sitter to pick her up.

Now I see two girls, about eight and eleven, who belong

to the mystery woman. They take Hannah's hands, help her wash up, then walk her out of the ladies' room to me.

"I saw you were having some trouble, so I thought I would help. I hope you don't mind," the woman says.

"No," I say. "You saved my life."

"She has a mind of her own, this one," the woman says. "No one is going to push her around."

"The mother's side of the family," I say.

The woman and her girls wave good-bye to Hannah.

"See you later, bye-bye, lady!" Hannah says.

I look down at my beaming daughter, the smallest kid among three bigger boys, and my heart melts. I have always been more short-tempered with Hannah than with her brothers. If Jared were having trouble in the potty I never would put so much pressure on him. I give Hannah less attention, less praise, fewer good-night kisses at bedtime. When she dresses by herself I hold her up as an example over the boys instead of just rewarding and appreciating her. I still have no idea why I have connected more slowly with Hannah, but I am ashamed of it. She is my only girl and she deserves her full share of attention, and I love her now, in this moment, more than ever.

"I made twenty-two poopies, Daddy," Hannah says, proudly holding up ten fingers.

"Wow—that's a good girl!" I say.

"Daddy, I'm thirsty," Asher says, pulling my shirt.

"I'm thirsty too," says Jared.

"I want lemonade," Asher says.

"Juice," Barak corrects.

"Uppie!" says Jared, clinging to my leg like seaweed.

"I want cookies and jelly beans and ice cream and *cake*," Hannah says, dotting each word in with her finger. "You *promised*."

SEVENTEEN

Transition Time

Four children fly through the air. Jared bounces off his Fisher-Price car bed and lands on the rug with his feet planted together—he always sticks the landing—then rolls into a series of tumbles. Hannah jumps up and down on her bed, a doll in each hand, screaming at the top of her lungs and thrashing her head. Barak hops up and down with his bedcovers draped over him. Asher balances on his bed frame and whips pillows at the other three.

Jared was up at 5:50 this morning, pushing a Barney puzzle in my face. I really need to segue this day into Daddy time.

The triplets are three and a half now, Asher six, and they understand they are misbehaving. But they are over-tired and once they quiet down they will be asleep within seconds. One good finesse and I'm home free. Tomorrow morning they will be exhausted, Barak will cry for TV time, Asher will be late for school, and Jared, the little Super-man, will be up again by 6:00 A.M.

When I wake up in the morning I am behind schedule. It doesn't matter how organized I am, how hard I plan, how many corners I cut. I will be twenty-five minutes late all day long. Nothing short of a change in the laws of physics will allow me to catch up.

The kids would be asleep already if we split them up in separate bedrooms. The army barracks concept is Roni's idea.

"I want them to be close," Roni says. "This is their special time together. I want them to be best friends."

Roni and I are close to our respective siblings, but not close in that intense, Waltons-like way we wish for our kids. But who among our contemporaries fits the Waltons criteria?

"That's why I want to do it. I want them to be different," Roni says.

I start to say that the kids will make better friends if they are well rested, but I am trying not to say what I normally say these days. Roni works late. She's not home to struggle with bedtime, but neither is she here to enjoy it. If I complain about unrealistic theories I am forced to administer she will say she can quit her high-pressure job and we can live in the country in a tumbledown house and scrape by—like the Waltons. So I have the argument in my head, where it can do no harm.

And Roni is probably right. It doesn't matter if the kids get to bed late today if sleeping in close quarters brings them closer together for the rest of their lives. I wish Paul and I were closer, that we lived near each other, hung out at each other's houses, went to ball games, bickered and teased each other like kids. With my mom gone I am acutely aware of how separate my life is from my brother's.

I think back on all the times I let him down. When he was initiated into his college fraternity, I was working and didn't make the two-hour drive to surprise him. Another time Paul was visiting me at college and I ate magic mushrooms and left campus in a panic with a high school buddy, abandoning him. I wish I had spent more time looking out for him, and I don't want my kids to repeat this kind of mistake.

Roni needs her systems followed as much for the value of her logic as for the expression of her love by proxy. In this way, she is home even when she is not. Although she can be annoying in expressing her love via management fiat, I have not been sensitive enough to this basic need.

"Daddy!" Asher screams. "We have a problem!"

I hear screaming. This is not good. I don't even look at the time as I turn from my office and run into the mayhem.

The four kids strip off their clothes and bomb through the house, naked and laughing and screaming. Imagine a 1970s hard-rock band let loose in a new hotel.

I corral them in their bedroom, behind the security gate. They test the gate, throw themselves against it, try to jimmy it open. Of course they can climb over the gate easily. It is really just a symbolic gate now.

Book time is final transition between chaos and order. I step over the gate, pick out a book, and sit on the floor, waiting for them to settle down. Usually Jared or Hannah will hang on my back and look at the book, causing the others to drift over.

This is not happening tonight. The final reserves of energy must be expended in one final crescendo of action, as blankets, books, toys, and clothes are heaved over the security gate. Barak cackles with pride as he sends books and toys crashing over the second-floor banister. I scold him about mistreating our books. We don't throw books in our house. From the hallway I pick up the books as Barak heckles me.

"No, we're not throwing any books, Bubba," Barak says, with his bizarre Red Skelton voice.

"Hiya, Bubba," Hannah adds, as she dumps load after load of clean, folded clothes over the gate and onto the floor with workmanlike precision.

"Bye-bye, Bubba," Jared says, jumping rope with one of Roni's bras in powerful, graceful leaps. I stand back and watch as the activity level tornadoes up. I have locked them behind the gate in an official time-out. I cannot give them an additional time-out. No time-out exists within the time-out. This would violate the time-space continuum.

At some point I have to step in—a head is banged, a toy smashed, a finger stepped on—and they become dangerous, biting and pushing, poking and stabbing, with toys converted into weapons.

When I broach the gate they go berserk and scream "Daddy's coming!" and explode into a blur of naked running torsos with gangly arms and legs slicing and dicing through the room. They leap from the headboards of their car beds onto their mattresses, trampoline to the carpet, vault improbably through the air, a miniature Cirque du Soleil. Asher eggs them on. "Climb up there! Run away from Daddy!" he yells.

I will never understand how they produce this volume of energy. I took chemistry in high school and cannot comprehend how their intake of calories supports twelve unrelieved hours of turmoil. Are the bodies of children that much more efficient than adults? Is anyone studying children to see how this chemistry can be applied to parents, who fall asleep at the computer at 4:00 P.M., even after coffee and a low-fat bran muffin?

The New York Times, my TV show, the writing assignments I have pushed off, my laundry, all loom as far away as next year's vacation. The house is lit up like a Christmas tree, the garbage sitting on the back porch is being chewed through by animals, the garage is open to wayward bats, play date phone calls must be returned.

I escort them to the potty one by one. I don't know why I insist on making gestures destined to fail, and yet I do, hoping that one night they will simply forget to crush my plans. The negotiating, potty going, and teeth brushing continue for twenty minutes. Bedtime requires two dozen individual trips to the bathroom. I never imagined that algebra would actually come in handy.

Eventually I trick them into their PJs with a small bribe—another book, a word game, even, in desperation, the disingenuous promise of candy tomorrow—which I pray will be forgotten in the fog of a new day.

After more petty extortion—I give them their pen flashlights, let them flick the window fan on and off—I finally coax them into bed. They are weary but defiant.

"I want cookies," announces Hannah. Two more heads pop up from under the bedcovers, awakened, zealous.

"Cookie time!" shouts Barak.

"Cookie time in the house!" sings Jared, hands on hips, swaying up and back. "Wheeee!"

I look at Jared. Is his enthusiasm a pure expression of glee or does he have a deeper appreciation of how the cookie distraction can sabotage the entire bedtime procedure?

"Bedtime," I correct.

"It's cookie time," sings Asher, banished to the den to watch TV, make long-distance phone calls, start fires—anything but stir trouble up in here.

"Back," I warn, threatening the removal of Asher's privileges—TV, computer, treats.

Asher's mind spins as he calculates the losses and eyes the babies malevolently. Asher can whip them up into an electron-bouncing fury with just a few shouts. I see him fast-forwarding the tape of how this might play out. Finally, he senses something in me—anger or desperation—and leaves.

The triplets settle down under their covers. There are muted waves of low noise, the rustling of blankets, grabbing of stuffed animals, soft squeaking farts, moans and sighs and stretches.

Rocky clutches his yellow comforter and sucks his thumb. Jared, the most finicky of the triplets, kicks off his blue-and-red blanket.

"That's Asher's," Jared complains.

Now Hannah shoves an extra blanket to the floor. "That's Rocky's!" she screams.

Each bed has a unique set of sheets and blankets. They each have a small blanket, taken from their crib when they were babies, matching sheets and pillowcases, several larger blankets, and finally a comforter. Each bed has a unique combination of linens. If any blanket or sheet or pillow is mixed up, bedlam ensues.

The First Rule of Triplets: Everything must be different. While invisible to the casual observer, to three competitive toddlers such minute differences are crucial.

Now Barak begs for water. I'm not supposed to let them drink after 7:00 P.M., to assist potty training, but this seems sadistic. Death-row inmates get water after lights out.

Screaming and wailing erupt as Hannah demands her share of water.

"It's just water!" I say. "Don't fight over water!" Of course they fight over water. They are three and a half years old. They fight over the Styrofoam peanuts used in packing boxes. "You're fighting over garbage," I say, as they tear into each other like brides at a bridal sale. They don't listen. Someone has a bigger handful of Styrofoam peanuts and the universe is all out of balance.

Hannah's hypervigilance over food and beverage dispensation amazes me. She will be denied not one drop, not one crumb. If Jared were eating dirt in the front yard with a teaspoon, she would head straight for the tablespoons.

Jared asks for the seltzer, which sets off another series of frantic negotiations. Volumes of water and seltzer must be compared, studied, adjusted. They attack my competence to perform measurements and criticize my methodologies.

The Second Rule of Triplets: Everything must be equal. These two directives must balance seamlessly, without canceling each other out.

It is well past 10:00 P.M. now. The babies rub their eyes, fighting sleep. Various schemes and scams are attempted. They want to call Mommy in the office, show me their art projects, go outside and check for storms on the horizon. Asher, who I watch carefully, is temporarily absorbed in his book in the den.

"There's a ghost in my bed," says Rocky.

"A ghost!" says Hannah.

They watch *Scooby-Doo*. I worry it will destroy their brains, hurt their college admissions, but I watched it faithfully, and I was nine or ten.

"Give the ghost a drink of water," says Jared.

"What if the ghost *kills Daddy*?" says Asher.

"Ghosts don't kill our daddy!" protests Hannah.

"You're very, very bad!" agrees Rocky. This leads to a round-robin of accusations and counteraccusations. Asher joyfully responds to each charge with an absurd counter charge—you have ice cream in your nose, a whale is going to bite your foot, your bed is full of invisible huffenfuevels.

I pick Asher up and carry him into the den, warning him with my not-kidding-now face that enough is enough. He takes it in stride. His eyes say he knows I'm putting on the tough-guy act.

Finally Hannah passes out and her little snores saw through the room. Rocky sucks his thumb, rolling around furiously. He corkscrews around his car bed, his extremities colliding with the wall, the radiator, the side rail. Rocky gets more exercise sleeping than I get in a week at the gym.

"I want to go to the big bed," says Jared. He whines, arms thrust up, waiting for me to pick him up. The Scammer is scamming.

I tickle Jared. He hides his face, but I know he is smiling under the angry wails.

"My tummy hurts," Jared says, switching tactics.

"Do you need to go to the potty?" I say.

"No. I just want to go to the big bed," Jared explains.

"Don't make a poopie in the big bed," offers Asher.

"*I don't make poopies in the big bed or anywhere!*" Jared says. Then he bursts out crying, heavy, fearsome tears. I pick Jared up and he clings to my neck. He is so strong, I feel him constrict my jugular vein.

Hannah wavers in and out of sleep. No advantage may be given, no favoritism shown. If I take even one half-step toward the door, Hannah will awaken with ferocious, howling contempt.

I rock Jared back and forth, trying to restore the blood flow to my brain, and inch toward the gate. I have one leg over when Hannah rises, screaming murder. I run down the hallway and drop Jared on the big bed, where he dives into the pillows. As I turn to leave I see, from the corner of my eye, the triumphant smile plastered across Jared's face. I am the fiddle and he the fiddler.

I add Hannah to the big bed, separating her from Jared with a pillow barrier. Asher has turned on the TV in the den. I hear him click it off when I stick my head in. He hides the remote under the seat cushion, smiling at me innocently with his best what's-the-matter? face.

I have vivid memories of my mother tucking me into my bed when I was a little boy, maybe three or four. I remember her standing in the doorway and smiling at me as I went through a very specific nightly ritual.

"Good night!" I said.

"Good night," my mom said.

"Sleep tight!" I said.

"Sleep tight," she said.

"Watch out for bed bugs. Sleep on your back, or your stomach, or any side you want," I said. I repeated a litany of bedtime-related freedoms and privileges. I remember my bedtime as quiet and peaceful and loving, my mom watching over me, vigilant and omnipresent. The peaceful memories last until the age of eight or nine, when I began to read *Ripley's Believe It or Not*, ghost stories, books about voodoo and the occult and Satanism, and scared myself silly. My favorite author was Edgar Allan Poe. For years I watched Rod Serling's *Night Gallery* and slept with the lights on. But I loved scary stories, so it was worth it.

I remember bedtime as warm and peaceful. I want my kids enveloped in that same bubble of serenity, but the current bedtime situation prohibits this. I tell myself that's how it is with four kids. They are bonding, cutting loose, enjoying the party.

I return Jared and Hannah to their beds and check my e-mail. A few minutes later I shut the bedroom light. The triplets are sleeping, cheeks red, arms and legs hanging over the sides of their beds. I straighten them out, re-cover them, tuck them in—the first of many such re-covers and tuck-ins I will conduct before dawn.

The house is strangely quiet. I stand at the door to the room, a buzz in my ear from the lack of sound. The quiet is alarming.

At the end of a long day I am glad they sleep together. I want them to be best friends when they grow up. I want them to live close to one another, drop by unannounced for dinner, raise their children as one large unruly group, butt in on each other's personal lives. I want them to have family meetings and discuss who is having a problem and needs help. I want them to finish each other's sentences.

Tomorrow night, when they bounce off the walls and ignore me in their delirium, I will be tired and frustrated, but this is the life they should have. I hope they look back and remember all the fun.

Now Asher begs for treats, books, games, TV, computer time. He remembers school projects that require emergency attention, play dates that need scheduling, a hundred semilegitimate stonewalling activities. We read for fifteen more minutes.

"It's ten-thirty," I say. "Time to brush teeth."

Asher casually wings his toothbrush, coated with Rugrats toothpaste, across the room. When I pick him up, he goes limp, like a nonviolent protestor. He smiles as I carry him through the war zone of the darkened bedrooms and into the bathroom. Along the way he reaches out and grabs every doorframe, every light switch, every open closet door, to knock me off balance.

Finally Asher is in bed, teeth brushed, kissed and hugged, covers adjusted.

"Can a black hole eat the sun?" Asher says.

"That's a good question," I say. "Let's discuss it tomorrow."

"If the first person on earth was a baby, who took care of it?" he says.

This catches me short. Where does he come up with these things?

"Tomorrow," I answer.

"You're so mean!" Asher sobs. He is exhausted. I sit with him, talking softly, as he drops off to sleep.

It is 10:55. I take Barak to pee in his sleep, because he cannot make it through the night. When I carry him, he pats me on the back in his sleep. I stuff dirty clothes in laundry bags, start the laundry, empty garbage, wash milk cups and plates and bowls, turn off lights, and take out the garbage. I empty and reload the dishwasher, warm up dinner, turn on the 11:00 local news.

The phone rings. Roni says she'll be home around 12:15.

"How's the tuna?" I say. Roni laughs. At work she orders the same dinner five nights a week—tuna tataki, medium rare, with rice and seaweed salad.

I recite outtakes from the day's highlights until she puts me on hold. There is a problem with the lawyers on the other side of the deal. There is a tie-up on the FDR Drive. Did I remember to RSVP for the—

Now there is screaming: Jared's voice, escalating with my delay. He will want water, potty time, the big bed, a book that has been missing for days. Another long night begins.

"I have to go back to work," I say to Roni. This is our little joke. Sometimes she teases me that I have it easy at home, like Florence Henderson in a fluffy fabric softener commercial, but I know she appreciates my end of the deal. We hang up and I nuke my unfinished cup of coffee.

"I'm coming," I yell, as another voice emerges— Hannah's. The cries melt into an angry, demanding chorus. "I'm coming," I yell, but they cannot hear me over their own wall of sound.

EIGHTEEN

The Value of Baseball Cards

Asher stands at the baseball plate, the batting helmet hanging lopsided on his head, blinking nervously at the coach. He swings at a low pitch and misses. In first grade baseball, kids are not allowed to strike out, a good rule, even if several times each game some poor kid is forced to take sixty or seventy doomed whacks before the coach mercifully nicks the ball off the fat end of the bat and into the infield dirt.

Asher knocks the second pitch down the third base line and reaches first base through a catalogue of errors, his face unsmiling, lips clenched. I unconsciously hold my breath. Asher is an average player playing at average skill level in the tight belly of the suburbs where average is a pornographic word. The sons of the three volunteer coaches play first, second, and third base in clannish rotation, fielding magnificently and mechanically pounding the ball into the outfield. Each boy has enjoyed devoted backyard drilling with his coach dad. I smile at the thought of these kids committing thousands of hours to learn the intricacies of bunting and stealing and split-fingered fastballs when the closest they will ever come to a career in professional sports is writing off their sky box as an un-reimbursed business expense. But I am also jealous of the hard-earned athletic skills and the dedicated father-son drill time. It worries me that Asher and I miss the luxury of quiet practice time, even though he wiggles out of whatever baseball practice I suggest. Baseball is not his sport; he chafes at playing in the games and barely tolerates practice. He is naturally gifted at soccer, plays aggressively, and follows the soccer schedule without complaint.

My happiest childhood memories are the warm spring and summer afternoons playing Little League ball, the fat slow kid who could hit deep. I looked forward to each game for days, the ritual of suiting up, watching the opposing pitcher throw, waiting for my turn at bat. Today is a warm Saturday afternoon in June 2001, and even though Asher could take it or leave it, I couldn't be happier.

The triplets are four and a half now and Asher is seven. Jared runs barefoot from the playground behind the baseball diamond and grabs my hand. He wants to demonstrate some cool move on the playground equipment. When I ask Jared where his sandals are, he laughs at me with the indulgent impatience of a fourteen-year-old whose dad wants to discuss trends in hip-hop.

In the playground Jared scrambles across a long S-shaped monkey bar and flips himself down to the platform at the end. What was difficult a few months ago is now easy for him, and he flashes that killer smile. Sometimes I fast-forward to him as a tan, hard-bodied sixteen-year-old boy lazily waxing his surfboard on a hot summer day, ignoring the phone calls of starstruck teenage girls. Even his teeth are straighter and whiter than mine ever were. I give Jared a hug and he squeezes my face between his two strong hands.

"You're the bestest daddy I ever seened," Jared says, intentionally misspeaking.

Now Hannah follows. While a few pounds heavier than Jared and an inch shorter, Hannah has tremendous arm strength. She climbs across easily but fumbles at the end because she starts laughing. "I can see your boobies," she says to me. "Your big fat hairy nipples." Jared and Asher scream with laughter, and Hannah, cracking herself up, falls from the bars like an overripe coconut.

Barak swings from the first few bars and looks at me. "Daddy, I'm falling," he says, hanging dramatically by one wobbly arm. I reach for him but he lets go and hits the sand with a whump. He sprawls out on his back and folds his arms across his chest.

"I'm dead," Barak says. His imitation of a dead person is ruined by his twisted smile. When I pick Barak up he tells me I have a crab on my head.

Jared and Barak stop to pee on a large oak tree. They love to pee outdoors and wiggle their rear ends in the air as if tree-peeing were an Olympic freestyle event. Hannah looks at me woefully. "I know, I know," I say.

The kids methodically demolish the cereal bars, Yoo-Hoos, apples, and crackers. Barak hands me the cell phone and tells me to order pizza. "Now!" Barak barks, bent over at the waist, wagging a finger at me. Is he joking or on the verge of a tantrum?

Jared wraps his arms around the back of my neck and makes me walk around the field as he dangles by an iron grip, unbreakable except for a tickling attack.

Barak approaches a mom from the other team and informs her she has a porpoise on her head, which he pronounces "purpose."

Hannah stares at two older girls playing with dolls, telepathically pleading with them to include her in big-girl world.

Asher waits for his at-bat and tosses dirt balls with another kid. I tell him to keep his baseball bat back and off his shoulder when he is up to—

"Daddy!" Asher interrupts, in a furious whisper. "You're bothering me! Go away!" Asher is much more rebellious and combative at home than ever before. We are happy he wants his independence but need to modify his disrespectful tone.

Jared jumps on me and hangs on my back as I pack up our stuff. Hannah tries to pull my shorts down, cackling maniacally. Jared tells Hannah to put leaves and branches down my pants. Barak holds my cold, half-finished coffee cup up over his head, threatening to douse himself. "Oh, no!" Barak says, dancing up and down. "Oh, no, the coffee is going to make a terrible gassy spill!"

Liza, the friendly mom who invited me to join her book club, laughs at all this, and says, "I was talking to Judy, and we couldn't decide whether you still like doing this job. The triplets seem like so much work."

I laugh. My creative writing career is dead. My job prospects are grim in the depressed New York media market. Roni is reaching the end of her rope at work and has started telling me to think about driving a limo or selling stereo equipment. We're broke and may not be able to keep the new house. The unanswered questions of how and why my mom died worm away inside me, because the autopsy failed to determine a cause of death. I don't know if the autopsy was even impartial.

In my mind I replay all the mistakes Paul and I made dealing with the doctors and the hospital, all the incompetence and bad medicine, all the alternate paths we could have taken. And then I replay the previous twenty years and berate myself for all the squandered opportunities to spend more time with my mom, all the trivial nonsense that kept me too occupied to see her, the holidays and birthdays that I foolishly let slip away. And she never once complained that I could do more. I should have done so much more. I wasted so much time.

But my time with the kids is pure playtime, an alternate universe from the worry-poisoned planet of adulthood. And this moment, with three kids goofily terrorizing me and another one smiling from the on-deck circle—approving the attack in progress by his troops—is better than I ever dreamed when I was in my twenties and searching for the meaning of life, which turned out to be a trick question.

Barak is two inches taller than Hannah and an inch or so taller than Jared. He has pale skin, thin blond hair, and freckles splashed across the middle of his face. Strangers often claim he looks like Asher. Rocky is the most complicated personality. Like Asher, he is an object fetishist and collects dozens of small, meaningless items in his own special box under his bed. Like Asher, Barak's collection of junk outgrew the first special box and required deployment of a secondary special box. Barak will wake in the middle of the night to ask about his magic wand or finger puppet or little plastic thingamabob. At any one time I am mentally tracking ten or fifteen small items for Barak across the three junk-swept floors of our house. Barak loves animals and insects and chases bunny rabbits and squirrels and summer fireflies. If we see a spider or fly in the house he will be furious if I try to kill it. "You can't kill living things because you're not God! You're just a daddy!" Barak will yell.

Barak is still exploring his feminine side. He loves to play with Barbies and requested a Barbie cake at his fourth birthday. He owns a pair of plastic high-heeled shoes—after screaming in jealousy over Hannah's pair—which he enjoys wearing around the house, often with glittery accessories. Sometimes Roni and I look at each other and wonder if this means anything. When I ask Barak what he wants to be when he grows up, he says, a mommy.

"But you're a boy," I say. "Aren't you going to grow up and be a daddy?"

"Sometimes I can be a girl if I'm not a boy that you're not a boy because you don't know what I'm saying I can be a boy or a girl tomorrow so what's your business?" Barak replies, eyes bulging with righteous indignation.

Barak is still the laziest kid and easily manipulates me into helping him get dressed, carrying him into the house from the car, and cleaning up his messes and spills. He is also our most dedicated TV addict. On the rare evening I go to the movies alone and Roni stays home with the kids, I usually find Barak wide-awake at 2:00 A.M. watching the Cartoon Network and Roni snoring on the couch next to him. When I turn off the TV he cries out, "Just one more minute! Please!" I put him on my lap and I give him his one more minute, because it will save me twenty minutes of his crying, pleading, and misbehaving. Sometimes one minute can be the best investment of a long day.

Barak is extremely affectionate and loving. Teachers and

relatives and family friends rely on Barak to fill any hug deficits. Barak hugs friends and teachers and the bus driver on a school trip. At night Barak asks me if I can sleep in his bed. When I tuck him in he puts my open hand on his pillow and lays his face on it. After the lights are finally turned off Barak hugs me tightly, and says, "I love you more than the universe and the stars and space and the whole world and the *contidents* and the trees and all the peoples and their heads and the bones in their heads. I love you this much, Daddy." Barak has his yellow baby blanket in his sights or knows its exact location at all times.

Jared's magnetic personality and self-confidence grow with every month. He is more naturally athletic and graceful than any family member going back one hundred years, and it is impossible to take an unflattering snapshot of him. When we take a hike with another family and encounter a fallen tree, all the kids line up to walk along its length. Two kids hold hands with a parent and stumble across. Asher falls off in the middle. Hannah struggles across, arms swinging wildly. Barak leaps off dramatically. But Jared walks along the tree as if walking down a hallway, his arms at his sides. Jared does perfect cartwheels. He has so little body fat that he starts shivering the minute he steps out of the bath. I can see the cuts on his delts and lats already. Jared has tremendous mental concentration and will work on an art project for an hour, coloring meticulously. Jared is still the neatest eater—just like when he was six months old—and the pickiest about wrinkles in his clothes. He always maintains the cleanest hands and face. Yet somehow he enjoys letting loose with window-rattling fake burps.

Jared still whines the most, has the most hair-trigger

crying response, and scams the most turns in the big bed. He is afraid of dogs. He can be curious and fearful at the same time. When a thunderstorm breaks out at bedtime Jared wants to know if the thunder is going to get them. Can the thunder come into the house? Is the lightning going to come through the windows? When I explain how a storm works Jared thinks it over for a minute, and then says, "Oh." Jared goes through a changing series of bedtime tuck-in rituals, from telling bad knock-knock jokes to grabbing my face and rubbing our noses together while laughing in a mad scientist's voice. Jared is also extremely affectionate with friends and family. He calls one of the girls in his Montessori class his "lovey" and says he is going to marry her and have babies. In the afternoon he breaks into my office to tell me he loves me and that I am the bestest daddy in the whole world, which he mispronounces, like Bugs Bunny, "woild."

Hannah plays with dolls and looks beautiful in a party dress but will never be a girly girl. She snores, guards her food like a prison lifer, and interrupts bath time with explosive farts. She is by far the most temperamental child. Between the ages of two and a half and three and a half she would literally scream nonstop for an hour when angry. During public tantrums Roni and I both feared being arrested for child abuse. The screaming has subsided, but Hannah still holds grudges for days and will give Roni the silent treatment until Roni goes bananas. We both tremble with fear over her teenage years.

But Hannah is the most independent. She dresses and undresses by herself seven days a week and picks out her own clothes, tossing my wardrobe selection back at me as if I were an idiot. She works on jigsaw puzzles relentlessly until completed, and attacks art projects with the same single-mindedness. Hannah loves to discuss bodily functions and body parts and thinks nothing of peppering a conversation with "penis" and "vagina." Hannah loves putting on makeup and hosting tea parties but she is tough as nails and never backs down from a fight, even with Asher. Sometimes I find Asher running around the kitchen island, trying to evade Hannah who, in her wrath, attacks unstoppably, like Jason Vorhees from the horror movies. Hannah began to read whole words before Jared and Barak and will busy herself with books for hours. Her favorite activity is a game where she is the pretend mommy, Jared the pretend daddy, and one of her dolls the pretend baby.

Unfortunately, this game often leaves Barak out of the equation. Hannah and Jared's unusual closeness often precludes Barak, a problem Roni and I secretly debate until Asher overhears us one day and scolds Jared and Hannah the next time a fake-family game begins.

"Barak is part of this family!" Asher screams.

Now Barak is wise to the controversy. "They're not letting me be part of this family," Barak moans, breaking in to my office to complain about Jared and Hannah.

And yet the closeness of Jared and Hannah reinforces Barak's individuality. In the middle of the first year of nursery school the teachers shock us with the information that Barak is the class leader, both in volunteering for projects and directing other children in activities. We did not see that twist coming.

The four kids play unsupervised for an hour or more now, moving from singing and dancing to chaotic chasing and fighting games to spying and surveillance exercises to board games with the rules wildly rewritten. Or they may fight every two minutes over the provenance of toys or the unfairness of a comment or some itching grudge. Usually these fights are resolved with a minimum of effort, but their ability to torment each other has grown more sophisticated and brutally effective. Buttons can be pushed, tantrums provoked, with a single, knowing glance.

In the car one day Jared and Hannah are talking and suddenly Hannah says she is not listening anymore. This is a favorite all-around torment. Hannah sings, "I can't hear you!" and claps her hands over her ears as Jared tries to talk to her. I patiently explain to Jared that if he ignores Hannah she will get bored and stop.

"No, she won't," offers Asher.

"Shhh," I say.

"I am ignoring Hannah, but she keeps pointing at me," Jared says.

"If you're ignoring her, then you can't see her pointing at you. She's invisible," I explain.

"But she's right next to me," Jared says.

"But that's what ignoring someone means," I explain. "You have to pretend she's not there."

"I can see her just fine," Asher says.

"I can't hear you!" Hannah yells.

"I am pretending she's not there, but she's teasing me," Jared says.

"She can't tease you if you don't let her," I say. "Just pretend she's not there and you can't hear her."

"No," Jared says, crying. "You make her stop!"

"She's just talking," Asher says. "People talk all the time."

"I can't hear you!" Hannah cackles.

"I'm being good, right, Daddy?" Barak says. "Big fat smelly Daddy."

· · ·

For years, Roni and I quibbled over child-rearing and household-operating issues like warring Afghan factions. But now we have made peace with our differences and even find comfort in them. When I serve ice cream to the kids, I see Roni looking at the bowls, waiting to see what will happen, and she sees me watching her, and then we both laugh, a wordless conversation. Our creative tension serves the children well.

We never say the words out loud, but have begun to accept each other's grievous limitations, along with the fact that we will not evolve much more as we age, except to become weirder and pricklier and more domestically challenged.

One Saturday Roni runs out the front door to make an impromptu tile-shopping excursion with Marla. I follow her onto the front lawn and argue that she is wasting her time, because we can't afford to renovate our bathroom and I was planning to clean out the garage. I have been chasing the four kids since 7:00 A.M. and am waiting to make the handoff.

Roni looks out the window of Marla's car, her feelings bruised. Her "one-hour" shopping trips with Marla often turn into mysterious all-day adventures, what with tag sales and the liquidator's warehouse store and the inevitable Chinese lunch buffet. This is her once-a-week girl time.

"If you don't want me to go, I won't go," she says.

Her face sags with disappointment, and I stand in the weedy, uncut grass, wondering what the hell I am doing. I send them on their way.

I chafed under Roni's bossy and critical nature for years,

yet now, here I am, insinuating that she prefers shopping over taking the kids to the playground. The harsh truth is that Roni is more accepting of my failed writing career than I am of her quirky and offbeat maternal sensibilities, which makes me a hypocrite.

Roni's influence on the children is highly visible. We can take the four kids to any nice restaurant or formal dinner party because Roni trained them in table manners, to sit still until the end of a meal, to be polite, to say please and thank you. (A sign on the dining room wall says Please and Thank You.) Roni got them off the potty before their third birthday. The four kids run/walk two miles around the high school track every Saturday with her, earning toys from the ninety-nine-cent store for finishing their laps. They do math and reading problems to earn Goldfish cracker snacks. Asher must read two chapters in his C. S. Lewis book to earn a night's sleep in the big bed. Roni organizes them to bake cookies and cakes and pies, to plant flowers and tomatoes and pull out weeds, to paint the outside benches, to bag up garbage. The triplets attend gymnastics class, and Roni harbors a schoolgirl fantasy that one of them might go to the Olympics someday. I tease her about being a stage mother, but I also thrill to the fact that she puts no limits on what the kids might achieve.

I show the kids how to play fair, take turns, and wear underwear on their heads. I teach the importance of hugs and kisses and swinging through my legs. I show them how to be funny and find the best spaces in hide-and-seek and not to worry when toys go missing or someone eats the last minimuffin or Asher calls them a fart-butter butt. I explain that monsters exist only on TV shows and in the movies. "We know, Dad, we know—God," says Jared. I cook their favorite foods and watch with delight as they chow down and gossip and argue and ask me to explain why all tigers are cats, but not all cats are tigers. When I try to explain the logic, Barak owls his eyes at me angrily, and now I am laughing and dropping pancakes on the floor and Jared is holding his belly and Barak is white-hot with anger at my misperceived insult, and then he is punching me and the kids are screaming and suddenly Barak is laughing too and I am holding him as he throws crazy wet dog licks at my neck and I am lost in the purest fog of bliss.

Within a year of losing my mom, my friend Rose Caruso died after a long, bitter battle with ovarian cancer, at forty-seven; my grandmother died at ninety-seven; and my first cousin Alex died at thirty-three after finally coming into his own as a doctor. Each funeral required driving on the New Jersey Turnpike, and I found myself staring out numbly at the exit signs so familiar from my childhood, but now so strange, wondering. *How did I get here, with this marriage, these children, this life? How did I marry the wrong person for the wrong reasons and end up with such a wonderful family? What if I had moved to Los Angeles when I was twenty-seven to pursue my comedy writing and never met Roni? What if I had accidentally erased her voice mail? Was there really any order in life besides wishful thinking?*

"It's not fair," Barak says one day, out of the blue, as we are walking to the playground. "God can see us, but we can't see God."

. . .

When I looked back over old family pictures, it seemed strange that I had few explicit memories before the age of nine, just fragments—we buy our beagle, Humphrey, when I am five, I get stitches in my head when I am six, Paul cuts open his rear end on a rusty slide when I am seven, some kids steal my banana-seat bike when I am eight. But these flashes of light could not illuminate who I was. Was I a happy kid? Who was my best friend? What was my favorite dinner? My dad was clueless. The answers are gone now.

Like most mothers, mine wrote the story of my life. (And, like most sons, I took her for granted, like the air I breathed, assuming she would always be around.)

She did not literally write the story of my life—as in a book or a diary—but she wrote it by being there every day. She watched as the person I know myself to be emerged from the primordial sludge of baby fat and spit and gurgling confusion. In the arrogance and self-absorption of youth, I was the misunderstood writer and she was the nice little mommy who always believed in me and had something positive to say, but could never understand my infinite complexities. Did other people ever fantasize about traveling back in time to slap themselves in the face?

At bedtime one night, Asher and Barak suddenly demand a story about Grandma. I am used to these inexplicable bursts of curiosity about my childhood, my mom, death, and God. Luckily, one story sticks out in my mind, the coffee story, my mom's favorite.

When I was ten or eleven months old, I would watch my mother drink coffee in the morning. I called it "gushee," which rhymes with tushie.

"No, it's coffee," my mom would say.

"Gushee," I said back.

"Try saying 'cough,' " my mom said.

" 'Cough,' " I said.

"Now say 'eee,' " my mom said.

" 'Eeee' " I said.

"Good. Now say 'cough-eee,' " my mom said.

"Gushee," I said.

The kids ask to hear the story over and over again, especially Asher, who retells it, with improvisational embellishments, after I leave the bedroom.

When Roni gets the kids dressed in the morning, I show her which pants are too short for Barak, which shirts are too tight to fit over Jared's head, what outfits Hannah refuses to wear, which socks the boys fight over. If she serves them breakfast I remind her to check the chart to see who gets the "golden spoon." If we have a baby-sitter, I remind her that Jared must have his feet tucked underneath his blanket and Barak must be taken to pee no later than 11:05 P.M.

To spend every day with them, to index their needs and choices and intolerances and dreams and sudden, inexplicable changes in taste, to oversee all the mundane intricacy of their days, I write their stories. One day I hope they will ask to hear them.

.   .   .

Barak and Asher karate fight even after a dozen warnings to stop. Jared jumps from the Naugahyde club chair onto the sectional couch, an acrobatic leap of some three feet. He narrowly misses Hannah each time, smiling the smile of the football captain who has just given a flying wedgie to a bench-sitter. Hannah screams at the top of her lungs but refuses to move, kicking and punching me when I try to remove her from harm's way.

Instead of raising my voice, I retreat and leave them five minutes of unsupervised mayhem. Gradually, slowed by bumped heads and scratched arms and pinched cheeks, they realize I have disappeared. When they search me out to complain about their mistreatment I sit on the floor of their bedroom, quietly removing the four special boxes from underneath their beds.

Waves of tears and lamentations engulf me. "No, not my special box!" they scream. I calmly explain they must get in bed and lie down quietly, or all the special boxes will be moved into my closet for one day.

"But Hannah pinched me!" Barak yells, refusing to get into his bed.

"Daddy!" Jared shouts, pulling on my hand with all his weight. He wants to take me into another room to offer some private explanation.

"What happened to my dinner?" shouts Asher, who ate dinner and a snack. "You can't just send a kid to bed without dinner!"

The whining and complaining escalate. I carefully place the four boxes on top of the armoire, making sure none of them open and rain precious cargo down into the room.

Their red faces contort with anger. After more screaming and wailing, they climb into their beds, angrily flipping down their covers. I am sorry to see such pure unhappiness, but relieved to seize back control without raising my voice. They are overtired and need to go to sleep.

I take the four special boxes down and carefully replace them under their beds. They rub their eyes and sniffle as I cover them with their blankets, kiss them and hug them, and reassure them that the special boxes are safe and sound.

I sit on the floor and adjust the special boxes under the beds. I can only use the special-box-removal ploy so many times before the kids realize I will never be so cruel as to harm or permanently remove them. Instinctively, they will understand the special boxes hold more magic for me than for them.

Why are the special boxes so magical? At first I thought they were a reminder of my baseball card trauma. After creating Asher's special box, I vowed to save a selection of their toys and artwork and baby clothes so they could decide, as adults, if they needed them. Not that some junky Pikachu card will turn out to be the Mickey Mantle rookie card of 2053, but they will be able to look at some of their old treasures, and say: This was mine, this was my life, this was me.

My nostalgic obsession with baseball cards erupted out of the blue in 1991, three years before Asher was born, long before I even considered the meaning of fatherhood. Now the episode seems like a weird and inexplicable flashback to childhood, a place where someone looked after me always, my needs were easily met, my every at-bat was wildly cheered, and disaster was a *How and Why* book with a page ripped out. The baseball cards were an unconscious dream, a wish to travel back in time, to live life over again, to correct mistakes, to say things left unsaid, to change the future. And yet the meaning of this dream escaped me. The wisdom of my own subconscious was lost. My mom sat next to me and I looked right through her to fiddle with my poor old water-stained 1967 Roberto Clemente card.

The baseball cards were not really baseball cards. They were something else, something irretrievable, something that could never be found once lost, a warning I was too ignorant to see.

Today I remove dried-out candies and pieces of dismantled household appliances from Barak's special box. Hannah's special box has become a sprawling Barbie doll organization, with clothes and accessories everywhere. I continually expand Asher's special-box infrastructure and smile over Jared's precisely organized, minimalist holdings. I am happy sitting here on the floor of my children's bedroom, surrounded by their totems of happiness, listening to them dream. Their special boxes remind me of what was, what endures, and what matters above all.